T0305742

Biomarker Analysis in Clinical Trials with R

Chapman & Hall/CRC Biostatistics Series

Series Editors

Shein-Chung Chow, Duke University School of Medicine, USA
Byron Jones, Novartis Pharma AG, Switzerland
Jen-pei Liu, National Taiwan University, Taiwan
Karl E. Peace, Georgia Southern University, USA
Bruce W. Turnbull, Cornell University, USA

Recently Published Titles

Data and Safety Monitoring Committees in Clinical Trials, Second Edition
Jay Herson

Clinical Trial Optimization Using R
Alex Dmitrienko, Erik Pulkstenis

Mixture Modelling for Medical and Health Sciences
Shu-Kay Ng, Liming Xiang, Kelvin Kai Wing Yau

Economic Evaluation of Cancer Drugs: Using Clinical Trial and Real-World Data
Iftekhar Khan, Ralph Crott, Zahid Bashir

Bayesian Analysis with R for Biopharmaceuticals: Concepts, Algorithms, and Case Studies
Harry Yang, Steven J. Novick

Mathematical and Statistical Skills in the Biopharmaceutical Industry: A Pragmatic Approach
Arkadiy Pitman, Oleksandr Sverdlov, L. Bruce Pearce

Bayesian Applications in Pharmaceutical Development
Mani Lakshminarayanan, Fanni Natanegara

Statistics in Regulatory Science
Shein-Chung Chow

Geospatial Health Data: Modeling and Visualization with R-INLA and Shiny
Paula Moraga

Artificial Intelligence for Drug Development, Precision Medicine, and Healthcare
Mark Chang

Bayesian Methods in Pharmaceutical Research
Emmanuel Lesaffre, Gianluca Baio, Bruno Boulanger

Biomarker Analysis in Clinical Trials with R
Nusrat Rabbee

For more information about this series, please visit: https://www.crcpress.com/Chapman--HallCRC-Biostatistics-Series/book-series/CHBIOSTATIS

Biomarker Analysis in Clinical Trials with R

Nusrat Rabbee

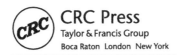

CRC Press
Taylor & Francis Group
Boca Raton London New York

CRC Press is an imprint of the
Taylor & Francis Group, an **informa** business

A CHAPMAN & HALL BOOK

CRC Press
Taylor & Francis Group
6000 Broken Sound Parkway NW,
Suite 300, Boca Raton, FL 33487

© 2020 by Taylor & Francis Group, LLC
CRC Press is an imprint of Taylor & Francis Group, an Informa business

No claim to original U.S. Government works

Printed on acid-free paper

International Standard Book Number-13: 978-1-1383-6883-5 (Hardback)

Visit the Taylor & Francis Web site at
http://www.taylorandfrancis.com

and the CRC Press Web site at
http://www.crcpress.com

Dedicated to

*Professor Emeritus **John A. Rice***

Department of Statistics

University of California

Berkeley, CA

Contents

Section I   Pharmacodynamic Biomarkers

Section II   Predictive Biomarkers

Section III   Surrogate Endpoints

Section V   Biomarker Statistical Analysis Plan

Foreword

Although I am not entirely sure what qualifies a person to write a foreword, I am incredibly grateful to have been asked to provide one for this book! Many published books are directed at academia, focused on theory, and sometimes prove helpful to students trying to master the subject. Books focused on the elegance of theoretical models have a place, but they may not aid the practicing statistician or the student that would like to become one. This book differentiates itself by focusing on the key inputs of biomarker analysis that can create great practicing statisticians. This book is focused on the practice of statistics. This book is a statistical lens for impacting clinical plans in the pharmaceutical industry. To illustrate the need and focus of this book, I want to draw the readers' attention to three key features: communication, understanding, and synthesis.

The first feature of this book is communication. This book has many graphical examples. Graphs are visual communication. Since many statisticians in early clinical development spend much of their study team time with non-statisticians, early development statisticians know succinct communication skills are a must. Without strong communication skills, a statistician may struggle to impact clinical studies and development plans. This communication will happen verbally and visually. A hard-won truth for the practicing statistician is if you cannot communicate your ideas to cross-functional team members, it often does not matter what statistical wizardry you can perform on data. A practicing statistician is only as impactful as their ability to communicate. While this book does not focus on verbal communication, it does teach about graphical communication. If you want to visually communicate biomarker data, this book will hone those skills. You may be tempted to skip over the visualizations to get to the meat of the analysis. Do not do it. Enjoy the visualizations for what they are, the first step in learning to work within cross-functional teams through visual communication techniques. Your career could depend on your communication skills one day.

The next feature of this book is the impact it will have on your understanding of the growing world of biomarker analysis. While it is impossible to cover every analytical innovation, this book will ground you in the most common aspects of biomarker data analysis. With the first three sections focused on pharmacodynamic, predictive, and surrogate biomarkers, this book will enable statisticians to quickly increase their biomarker analysis understanding. Not only is the book organized around these key areas, the subsections all focus on practical examples. Is your study preclinical or clinical? Is it in phase 1 or 3? You can quickly understand how to tackle these problems. You will also have enough of a foundational understanding to look for other techniques that are more recent. The organization and content of this book exemplify the structure thought needed to ensure biomarkers impact clinical development and you will have a better understanding through reading this book.

This book ends on a note about synthesis. In industry, communicating data is not enough. Analyses that highlight understanding will not get you there either. The communication and understanding need to be boiled down to enable clinical development teams to make stronger decisions than they could have previously. The section on combining multiple biomarkers drives us to think how information can be aggregated for decision making. This could have an impact preclinically, in early development or late. A practicing statistician will remain focused on driving stronger decision making. One promising area is combining data. The thought process needed to combine endpoints can change your biomarker analyses. A great place to begin this thinking is synthesizing biomarker information.

The world is awash in data. This volume of data will continue to increase. In the pharmaceutical industry, much of this data explosion has happened around biomarker data. Great statisticians are needed to derive understanding from these data. This book will guide you as you begin the journey into communicating, understanding, and synthesizing biomarker data. Good luck!

Jared Christensen
Biostatistics
Early Clinical Development, Pfizer, Inc.

Preface

This book is for statisticians who are working on biomarker data analysis in any and all phase of drug development. Nonstatisticians who are well versed in intermediate-level statistical theory and models used in clinical trial data analysis may use it as well. Knowledge of R programming language is presumed. Linear models, survival data analysis, multivariate models, probability theory, multiple comparisons, trial design, and statistical learning models are useful prerequisites. At least a master's degree level statistical knowledge will be required to get the best utility out of this book.

Objectives

This book reflects my experiences of the type of analyses conducted by statisticians working in biomarker data analysis in clinical trials. After spending more than a decade and a half in the drug and diagnostics development industry focusing on the analysis of biomarker, bioinformatics, and imaging data, it was time to write a book closely tied to the practice of statistics in biomarker analysis in drug development. This work would consist of mainstay topics in mathematics and computational statistics (such as joint likelihood methods or bootstrap methods), descriptive statistics, models encountered in analyzing pharmacodynamics, and predictive and surrogate biomarker data. Special attention is given to using R to generate user-friendly graphical displays of the results. The examples show the special significance of R, as well as the importance of data visualization in the industry. The examples will give the reader a taste of how modern statistics – combined with the power of R – can elucidate the effect of the drug being developed on the clinical outcome through the biomarkers. Given that the field is highly computational in practice and is based on mathematical statistics in principle, I assume that the student will have acquired the requisite theory in their academic training. Thus, this book can serve as a biomarker data analysis companion grounded in statistical theory.

Approach

Biomarkers in clinical development for drugs is becoming increasingly prevalent. In oncology, for example, the recent advances in immuno-oncology have utilized markers for immune cell response generously.

Some books do exist on this subject; however, they do not address the determination of cutoffs for a single predictive biomarker, or methods of visualizing the impact of biomarker on the efficacy endpoint, or combining biomarkers or surrogate endpoints.

Many existing resources are useful as statistics text books – typically with strong treatment of statistical issues; and many books focus on the clinical development context for biomarkers, which is necessary to understand why we conduct such scientific exploration in the clinic. Recently, there have been multiple books that have helped the readers understand the general methods and challenges in statistics behind modern-day drug development. This book aims to provide an introduction to biostatistics specifically in the context of biomarker data in clinical trials. It is an example-based approach to capture the main aspects of biomarker data analysis from preclinical to phase III trials. The examples show the wide variety of models needed for biomarker analysis that I have had the opportunity to use in my cumulative experience as an industry biomarker statistician. I have tried to capture the best practices for analyzing and visualizing biomarker data that are useful to biomarker scientists and clinicians.

I want to mention five key features of this book:

- First, the book is meant to serve as a reference textbook for biomarker data analysis for pharmaceutical industry statisticians or those who are interested in going into the field. Biomarkers are an integral, substantial part of many clinical development programs in oncology, immuno-oncology, autoimmune diseases, and psychiatric illnesses. The analyses considerations are distinct from primary and secondary efficacy endpoints and often dealt with lending supplementary evidence to the efficacy analysis of the drug. This book is not meant to serve as a book for diagnostic biomarker development, which discriminates between disease status, type, or severity. There are very good books that cover the statistical aspects of biomarkers in the diagnostics industry.

- Second, I divide the book into four main sections, (I) pharmacodynamic biomarkers, (II) predictive biomarkers, (III) biomarkers as surrogate endpoints, and (IV) combining a few biomarkers into a single composite measure. Section II contains concepts and R code for dichotomizing a continuous biomarker based on correlation with clinical response.

- Third, the approach I have taken is an informal dialogue with my audience where I will mention aspects of the clinical development program for each section in a chapter and focus on code snippets for practical demonstration of related analyses. R is overwhelmingly used by biomarker biostatisticians for the ease of tapping into the worldwide submission of complex packages in the language, as well as its wide use in graduate academic programs from where statisticians are graduating.

- Fourth, I do not cover statistical theory in this book; but I will provide the template for applying the theory in biomarker data by worked example. I will, however, give references to textbooks and to published papers for details of data sets or particular methods. There are two distinct advantages to this approach: (a) I am not writing yet another textbook on statistical theory, but rather referencing them for proper context for the student or the industry statistician; and (b) I am providing worked examples in R of the application of the theory using published or simulated data sets containing clinical trial data with biomarkers.

- Fifth, the phase of clinical development for each chapter will be discussed for context. What question needs to be answered? The context determines what type of statistical test will be performed and what type of visualization is useful. The context of the biomarker in clinical development program will be relevant and understandable to biostatisticians

- Sixth, I emphasize visualization of biomarkers, as this is important to explore how best to display one or several biomarkers changing over time to provide evidence of efficacy or target engagement or safety to the scientific and regulatory communities. Every chapter therefore has numerous examples on plotting using best practices in the industry.

Brief Outline

A brief outline of this book is provided below for the reader.

- In Section I, the topic of pharmacodynamic biomarker is covered from understanding mechanism of action to providing supplementary proof of efficacy. Statistical issues for biomarker statisticians cover the wide terrain of clinical studies. I cover specific biomarker-related topics in animal sacrifice designs, bioequivalence studies, and visualizing and modeling downstream longitudinal data showing support for proof of efficacy. Joint modeling of clinical outcome (survival data) and biomarker is included as special interest. The relevance of exploring such biomarkers through clinical trials is explained in the beginning of Section I. The objectives of analyzing longitudinally collected biomarker provide the important step of mechanistic understanding of the drug actions inside the human body which may serve as proxy for the presence/absence of clinical benefit.

- In Section II, the topic of predictive biomarker is covered. This is important especially in the time of precision medicine where a subset of patients with biomarker positive status may respond to the particular therapy being investigated. However, uncertainty remains about those who are biomarker negative. This is a huge area with many statistical developments; I focus on the cases where the subgroup is not clearly defined or the effect in the negative subgroup has not been ruled out. The chapters in this part deal with identifying a cut point (threshold) for a quantitative or semiquantitative biomarker, exploring sample size required for the biomarker positive and negative subgroups. Examples of considering the two subgroups are given in both the proof of concept and confirmatory trial settings. As a special interest topic, the seamless trial combining two stages – one exploring whether the treatment works only on the biomarker positive subgroup – and another confirming the effect on the positive and/or the overall population is included.

- In Section III of the book, the topic of surrogate biomarkers is covered. It typically takes multiple trials to establish a biomarker as a full surrogate for a clinical endpoint in a particular therapeutic area. Therefore, a meta-analytic framework for combining results from multiple trials are covered. In addition to establishing the correlation within the trial between the endpoint, the biomarker is discussed as well. Proportion of treatment effect is an important metric that has been used to establish CD4 cell count as a surrogate for AIDS/HIV clinical trials, and this has been introduced as a special topic of interest. Even if the biomarker does not get immediately filed as a surrogate endpoint, its utility in corroborating evidence ahead of, or in addition to, the approved clinical endpoint, is very useful. Statistical methods can help establish that utility and the sponsor of the trial can use that information for trial planning purposes.

- In Section IV of the book, the topic of combining a few continuous biomarkers into a single predictive measure of the clinical outcome is discussed. Regularized regression models are introduced with R code for the prediction and variable selection. Trees are also discussed, since they convey relationships between predictors and outcome variables in an intuitively meaningful to clinicians. As special interest, graphical models are discussed, as well as a popular graph regularization method, to find predictive association among biomarkers or clinical outcomes when $p \gg n$.

- In Section V of the book, a template for biomarker statistical analysis plan is introduced. This is an important tool in laying out the roadmap for the analysis of all biomarkers in the clinical trial. The amount and quality of forethought will maximize the gains from the biomarker analysis.

R Programming

A PC and a Mac were used to generate all the examples in this book. I have used R exclusively and have mentioned the specific packages used in solving the examples. However, there may be several alternative packages that may solve the same problem. It is left up to the reader to explore different choices. Graphs in R are generated by both regular plot() functions as well as functions in R library ggplot2. R programming and data visualization in R is rapidly evolving, giving more concise programming commands and informative displays. The general principles of presenting data in the right context through graphs remain the same. All the data and programming examples are available at the book's website at https://tinyurl.com/vnfw85s.

Acknowledgments

I am grateful to a number of people, institutions, and resources for making this book possible. I am indebted to David Grubbs for publishing this first edition. The universe of R package contributors, statistical theories behind the implemented packages, the numerous vignettes have been extremely useful in making these advanced models easily accessible to the readers. I acknowledge, Dr. Lianqing Zheng, who supported the book by diligently formatting the chapters, as made collating and annotating the examples and code such that they are accessible to the reader on the website (https:// tinyurl.com/vnfw85s). I appreciate the patience, persistence, and faith of my editors, publisher, and assistant in bringing this project to completion.

Author

Nusrat Rabbee is a biostatistician and data scientist at Rabbee & Associates, where she creates innovative solutions to help companies accelerate drug and diagnostic development for patients. Her research interest lies in the intersection of data science and personalized medicine. She has extensive experience in bioinformatics, clinical statistics and high-dimensional data analyses. She has co-discovered the RLMM algorithm for genotyping Affymetrix SNP chips and co-invented a high-dimensional molecular signature for cancer. She has spent over 17 years in the pharmaceutical and diagnostics industry focusing on biomarker development. She has taught statistics at UC Berkeley for 4 years.

Section I

Pharmacodynamic Biomarkers

1

Introduction

Biomarker development is a very active area in drug development for their utility in screening, diagnosing, monitoring disease, as well as for predicting treatment modulated clinical outcome. Of these, pharmacodynamic (PD) biomarkers are used from early phase human pharmacology stage studies to late phase studies to obtain pharmacological information of drugs interacting with the physical systems under study (e.g., heart, kidneys, central nervous system). Pharmacological *effects* of drugs on cells, organs, and systems are measured in animals in preclinical studies and in humans in controlled clinical experiments in the drug development process. The goal is to study drug characteristics for assessing target engagement and confirming mechanism of action (MoA). In precision medicine (especially in oncology), the MoA confirmation in humans is a key step in advancing the drug toward clinical development from preclinical development.

Biomarkers can be biological properties or molecules that can be detected and measured in parts of the body like the blood or tissue. Biomarkers can be specific cells, molecules, or genes, gene products, enzymes, or hormones. Complex organ functions or general characteristic changes in biological structures can also serve as biomarkers [1]. In early phase clinical trials, the drug manufacturer is focused on developing MoA assays for the drug. There is extensive literature about the development of MoA assays, as well as on developing other PD biomarkers, which measure further downstream molecular, biochemical, and physiological changes. Let us take an example of the latter type of PD biomarkers, specifically blood-based biomarkers. (i) In oncology, in order to study the pharmacologic effect of the drug on cancer tissues, an invasive biopsy of the actual tumor is usually needed. Current progress of science permits us to measure blood-based biomarkers of circulating tumor cells as alternative biomarkers of antitumor activity. (ii) In brain disorders, like Alzheimer's disease, blood biomarkers are less prevalent, since brain disorders may not have peripheral manifestation. However, blood and cerebrospinal fluid (CSF)-based biomarkers are presently an active area of research and development in neurology. (iii) In cardiovascular disease, hemoglobin A1c may be used as a PD/response biomarker when evaluating patients with diabetes to assess response to antihyperglycemic agents.

Several PD biomarkers over several phases of clinical development may be needed to constitute a complete picture of the drug's mechanism in the body from minutes to hours and days of drug administration [2]. The effort of developing assays and measuring the relevant biomarkers help drug development in the following ways:

- validating target engagement
- selection of optimal dose
- identifying potential early efficacy and/or safety
- potential identification of patient subgroup likely to respond from treatment with the drug
- help design combination therapies

Pfizer has defined three pillars of survival of a drug through clinical development in order to progress to phase III [2]. In order for the drug candidate to show potential efficacy in patients, it must demonstrate

i. exposure at the target site of action over a desired period of time
ii. binding to the pharmacological target as expected for its mode of action
iii. expression of pharmacological activity commensurate with the demonstrated target exposure and target binding

The evidence must be taken together in an integrated framework for decision-making. For pillar (i), since the drug concentration at the cellular level (target site of action) is usually not measured, pharmacokinetic (PK) concentration of the drug levels in plasma is taken instead. Taken together with the MoA PD biomarker(s) response as evidence of proof of mechanism (pillar ii), it is considered sufficient to continue through the drug development cycle. For pillar (ii), we measure one or more PD biomarkers to characterize the MoA and optimize dose selection. In the case of multiple drug regimen, drug–drug interactions must be understood (both synergy and antagonism) by means of more than one PD biomarkers [4]. For pillar (iii), a practical measurement of clinical benefit through a PD biomarker(s) is achieved in early clinical trial setting (phase I or II). Cartwright et al. [3] give an example in which the clinical outcome of interest is the long-term change in hemoglobin A1c and the PD biomarkers for assessing the benefit in the decreasing order of relevance are

- change in hemoglobin A1c at an earlier time point, for example, after 12 weeks of treatment, than the clinical endpoint time
- change in plasma glucose after 14–28 days
- change in other biochemical or enzymatic parameters after 1–7 days
- drug concentrations in the plasma (PK)
- information on hemoglobin pertaining to another drug in the same class that is already in the market

While the Proof of Mechanism (PoM) studies (pillar ii) seek to confirm that the drug engages its intended molecular target and alters the target function, Proof of Concept (PoC) studies (pillar iii) seek to link the molecular effect with the clinical response. The formal definition of PoC study is given as follows:

> POC is the earliest point in the drug development process at which the weight of evidence suggests that it is 'reasonably likely' that the key attributes for success are present and the key causes of failure are absent [3].

These studies need not be mutually exclusive. Often a PoM study is expanded in sample size to gather preliminary read outs on (PD assessments of) clinical response. Through early clinical phase studies (Phases 0, I a/b, and II a/b), the drug development program needs to establish both PoM (including optimal dose) and PoC of the investigational agent, as defined by the three pillars of success at Pfizer. If the MoA of the drug is already known and established, then PoC study can be the first step [4].

Statistical analyses are not only performed separately at each pillar but also to correlate the evidence between the three pillars. At the end, data from the early trials are often used to predict the probability of success for Phase II/III through clinical trial simulations.

The following table shows a rough sketch of the drug development process broken out by preclinical and clinical trials.

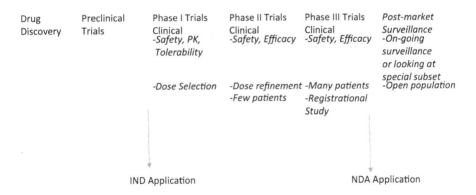

In the diagram above, *Drug discovery* stands for the highly scientific, high-throughput process for screening (HTS) many compound libraries, finding hits that are further reduced into leads. Various applications of statistics and computer science algorithms and robotics enable chemistry to guide the process to the selection of the final compound or set of compounds. We do not cover the statistical analyses of this process in this book.

Preclinical Trials aim to identify the best compound to take into clinical trials. Both in-vitro and in-silico testings of the compounds are carried out at this stage. The safety of the molecule is tested for toxicity in animals. When a promising candidate is found, the sponsor files for an Investigational New Drug (IND) application, along with all the preclinical data to the Food and Drug Administration (FDA). We cover the statistical analyses in a limited sense for pre-clinical trials in this Part of the book.

Phase I clinical trials study the PK/PD characteristics of the drug in human body. Dose and/or schedule selection is typically made in this phase where the maximally tolerated dose (MTD) is identified. We discuss a few statistical issues relating to evaluating PD biomarkers for the drug in later Parts of the book for phase I drug development.

Phase II clinical trials studies attempt to answer if the chosen dose (or dose range) and/or schedule shows treatment effect on the clinical outcome of the patient by comparing treated subjects with those on placebo or standard of care. In addition to randomized two-arm designs, Phase II trials may be a single-arm design, or may have multiple new treatments or doses.

Phase III clinical trials are conducted if Phase II studies are successful. These are registrational trials with two or more arms, consisting of multiple sites and a large number of patients. The studies are conducted for a new treatment in a well-defined population where the treatment and placebo/standard of care are administered to the patients in a randomized manner. We cover several topics of biomarker analyses in Phases II and III of drug development in later Parts of the book.

If the Phase III trial is successful in meeting the primary endpoint, then the sponsor can submit the New Drug Application (NDA) to the FDA for approval to market the drug in the United States.

Postmarket surveillance or Phase IV clinical studies are conducted in the open population of drug users. These data are used to answer additional questions about the product.

2

Toxicology Studies

Toxicology studies in animals are carried out very early in the drug development process. Designing and analyzing data from these toxicokinetic and
pharmacokinetic studies are part of the vast number of duties of nonclinical statisticians or biomarker statisticians. There are many statistical topics
involved in toxicology studies, and I will talk about a few *selected* topics (like
sample size calculations) to exemplify the use of R in solving these issues.

Rodent in-vivo toxicology studies are initiated and completed prior to
clinical PK studies in humans. Drug exposure is measured by the area under
the concentration × time curve (area under the curve (AUC)) or maximum
concentration (Cmax) at the expected peak concentration time (Tmax) [7].
See the following figure.

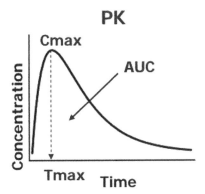

The clinical trial sponsor should consider the nonclinical safety/toxicological
data requirements outlined in ICH M3(R2) guidance of the Food and Drug
Administration (FDA) to design the appropriate nonclinical toxicology/
toxicokinetic studies to support a 'proof of concept' trial in humans.

2.1 Calculating the Number of Animals

Calculating the number of animals needed for the preclinical tox study
needs statistical guidance and input. For large animals, each animal is
usually sampled per time point giving rise to a complete design. For rats
and mice, we usually have *serial* sampling, where only one sample per subject is available, or *batch* or sparse sampling, where more than one sample

(but not the complete time course) is available from the animal. In the latter case, calculation of AUC and its standard error is complex.

Holder et al. [8] recap the three designs and the corresponding calculations for the three designs. First, the three designs are introduced in a tabular format below (Tables 2.1 through 2.3) for ease of depiction. The concentration at each time point is denoted by z.

When each animal is measured at each time point, estimation of AUC and its standard error are provided by Bailer and Nedelman et al. [5,6]. This is the case of complete design (Table 2.1). For the serial sacrifice design (Table 2.2), the Nedelman [6] method can be used for AUC estimation. However, for the batch design (Table 2.3) where the measurements on the same animals are positively correlated and each time point need not appear only in one batch, new methodology was necessary to calculate the variance estimator. I describe below the AUC method of estimation, particularly the one based on partial AUC.

TABLE 2.1

Complete Data Design

Times (t_j)	1	2	4	6
Weights (w_j)	1	1.5	2	3
Subject_i				
1	z_11	z_12	z_13	z_14
2	z_21	z_22	z_23	z_24
...	.	.	.	.
n	z_n1	z_n2	z_n3	z_n4

TABLE 2.2

Serial Sacrifice Design

Times (t_j)	1	2	4	6
Weights (w_j)	1	1.5	2	3
Subject_ib				
11	z_11			
21	z_21			
12		z_12		
22		z_22		
13			z_13	
23			z_23	
14				z_14
24				z_24

TABLE 2.3

Batch Design

Times (t_j)	1	2	4	6
Weights (w_j)	1	1.5	2	3
Subject_ib				
Batch 1				
11	z_111		z_112	
21	z_211		z_212	
Batch 2				
12		z_121		z_122
22		z_221		z_222

2.2 Partial AUC Method

Holder et al. [8] introduced *the partial AUC method* in this context, where batch b would investigate specific timepoints and the AUC estimate for treatment k would then be the weighted sum of the partial AUCs of the batches. Holder [8] introduces the formal notation for deriving the partial AUC method, which works for complete data, serial sacrifice, and batch designs.

Let k be the treatment doses, 1, ..., K; t be the time points of measurements from 1, ..., J; and $m_{k1}, m_{k2}, \ldots m_{kJ}$ be the mean responses for treatment k at each time point.

Then, $AUC_k = \sum_{j=1}^{J} w_j m_{kj}$, where the weights w_j are defined by the trapezoidal rule:

$$w_j = \frac{t_{j+1} - t_{j-1}}{2} \text{ for j} = 1,2,\ldots, J-1 \text{ and}$$

$$= \frac{t_J - t_{J-1}}{2} \text{ for j} = J$$

The AUC estimate for individual i with treatment k was summarized by Holder for complete and serial sacrifice designs. However, the partial AUC method was introduced as a novel method for estimating the AUC and its standard error for batch designs, which includes the complete and serial sacrifice designs as special cases.

2.2.1 Means and Variances

First, the partial AUC is created for subject i in batch b in treatment k as

$$p\_AUC_{kbi} = \sum_{j=1}^{J} w_j z_{kbij}$$

Second, the complete AUC for treatment k is defined as

$$\widehat{AUC}_k = \sum_{b=1}^{B} \overline{p\_AUC}_{kb}.$$

which involves the mean of partial AUC for all animals in batch b. Note that each animal contributed only one partial AUC to the equation above. For simplicity of notation, I have assumed that the number of animals in each batch is the same, as well as each batch has the same number in each treatment. However, this is not a requirement for the methodology.

Note there is an intraindividual correlation in the calculation of variance for p_AUC_{kbi}. The formula for standard error of the AUC estimate is given below:

$$\widehat{V}_k = \sum_{b=1}^{B} \frac{s_{kb}^2}{N_{kb}}$$

where the estimated variance of each p_AUC_{kbi} is $s_{kb}^2 = \frac{\sum_{i=1}^{N_{kb}} \left(p\_AUC_{kbi} - \overline{p\_AUC}_{kb.} \right)^2}{N_{kb}-1}$, with $N_{kb} -1$ degrees of freedom (N_{kb} is the number of animals in treatment k, batch b).

Assuming $N_{kb} = N_k$, we have $\frac{\widehat{AUC}_k - AUC_k}{\sqrt{\widehat{V}_k}} \to N(0,1)$. Holder also provides the degrees of freedom for the asymptotic Chi-square distribution of $\widehat{V}_k$. A pooled variance estimate of $\widehat{V}_k$ is also provided, since a single treatment group may have few observations at each time point and pooling variance estimates across treatment groups may sometimes be useful.

2.2.2 Contrasts

In Section 4 of their book, Holder et al. [8] derive the test statistics and linear contrasts for various hypotheses, including dose trends and proportionality. The linear contrasts make the comparisons between the mean AUCs of the treatment groups. For any contrast vector $[c_1,\ldots,c_k]$ such that $\sum c_k = 0$, the null hypothesis is distributed as central t. The degrees of freedom for the distribution of the test statistic is also given. When a large number of treatments are compared, the Dunnett's test is recommended.

TABLE 2.4

1st Example Sequence of Contrasts

Contrast	Reverse Helmert Codes	Detect the Endpoint of Response				
	Dose 1	Dose 2	Dose 3	Dose 4	Dose 5	Dose 6
Dose 1 vs Rest	5	−1	−1	−1	−1	−1
Dose 2 vs Rest	0	4	−1	−1	−1	−1
Dose 3 vs Rest	0	0	3	−1	−1	−1
Dose 4 vs Rest	0	0	0	−2	−1	−1
Dose 5 vs Rest	0	0	0	0	1	−1

TABLE 2.5

2nd Example Sequence of Contrasts

Contrast	Reverse Helmert Codes	Detect the Start Point of Response				
	Dose 1	Dose 2	Dose 3	Dose 4	Dose 5	Dose 6
Rest vs Dose 2	−1	1	0	0	0	0
Rest vs Dose 3	−1	−1	2	0	0	0
Rest vs Dose 4	−1	−1	−1	3	0	0
Rest vs Dose 4	−1	−1	−1	−1	4	0
Rest vs Dose 6	−1	−1	−1	−1	−1	5

We know that the omnibus F statistics from classic ANOVA does not distinguish between the means of treatment groups. So, contrast coding is used to compare means of treatment groups to one or more control groups.

Helmert codes are useful in assessing the dose level (or timepoints) at which a response stops or starts. The following are examples of codes for testing six treatment groups (doses) to find where the AUC for concentration starts or stops (Tables 2.4 and 2.5).

UCLA Statistics web page [9] states, 'Helmert coding compares each level of a categorical variable to the mean of the *subsequent* levels'. For more examples of implementation in R, the reader can visit the site.

2.2.3 R Code

The R code to implement the methodology described in Holder [8] is given below:

```
Y=read.csv(file.path(out,"/papers/part_I/AUC.
csv"),colClasses = "character")
```

```
W=Y[1,5:ncol(Y)] #weights
w=as.numeric(W)
B=table(as.factor(as.character(Y$Batch[-1])))
K=unique(Y$Dose_k[-1])
T=c(1,2,4,6,10,24)
z=matrix(NA,length(K),length(B))
v=matrix(NA,length(K),length(B))
for (k in 1:length(K))        #treatment
{
      for (b in 1:length(B)) #batch
      {
         data=data.matrix(Y[Y$Batch==b & Y$Dose_k==K[k],5:
         ncol(Y)])
         z.ibk=apply(data,1,function(x) sum(x * w,na.
rm=TRUE)) #partial AUC for animal i
         z[k,b]=mean(z.ibk,na.rm=TRUE)
         v[k,b]=var(z.ibk,na.rm=TRUE)
      }
}


#Partial AUC for each dose - sum over batches
AUC.hat=rep(NA,length(K))
AUC.hat=apply(z,1,sum)   #sum of partial AUC of batches
var.AUC.hat=apply(v,1,mean) #mean of partial AUC estimated
variances of batches
se.AUC.hat=sqrt(var.AUC.hat)
f=var.AUC.hat^2/(apply(v^2,1,sum)/(b^2*(b-1)))
Nbar.k=rep(18,length(f)) #average batch sample size
d=c(100,300,450,600,750,1000)
d.dot=(sum(Nbar.k * d))/(sum(Nbar.k))


#Plot the AUC +/= SE for each dose (treatment group)
df=data.frame(AUC=AUC.hat,SE=se.AUC.hat,Dose=K)
df$Dose=factor(df$Dose, levels=unique(df$Dose))
ymin=30
ymax=130
ggplot(df, aes(x=Dose, y=AUC.hat, group=1)) +
  geom_line() +
  geom_errorbar(width=.1, aes(ymin=AUC-SE,
  ymax=AUC+SE), colour="darkgrey")   +
  ylim(ymin,ymax)
```

The data are given in the chapter and entered into a.csv file where the first few lines are shown in Table 2.6.

The resulting plot of the Holder data of the mean AUC at each level and the corresponding confidence intervals are shown in Figure 2.1.

Obviously, the number of animals per batch will determine the width of the confidence interval. Since the larger AUC shows greater variability, you want to analyze the data in log scale and transform it back to original scale

TABLE 2.6

Data for Partial AUC Method

Subject	Batch	Dose_k	Weights (w_bkl)	1	1.5	2	3	9	7
		Times (t_i)		1	2	4	6	10	24
111	1	100 mg/kg		1.75			4.63		
112	1	100 mg/kg		2.2			2.99		
113	1	100 mg/kg		1.58			1.52		
121	2	100 mg/kg			3.03			3.34	
122	2	100 mg/kg			1.98			1.3	
123	2	100 mg/kg			2.22			1.22	

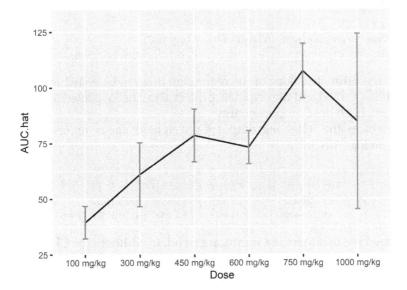

FIGURE 2.1
Holder data—Mean AUC and confidence interval.

before presentation. It appears that AUC is increasing with dose up to a certain point, and then the dose response curve may become a platueau. This is the case (monotonic dose response) where you may use the Helmert reverse coding to test contrasts of interest.

Since there are six doses, we can also perform linear regression with weights as the inverse of the standard errors of each $\widehat{AUC_k}$. We will need to make sure that we use log scale for computing the means and the standard

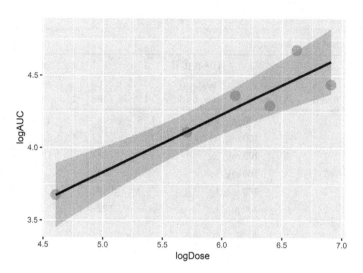

FIGURE 2.2
Holder Data—Regression between Log(Dose) and Log(AUC).

errors. The estimated slope of the regression line can be tested for $H_0 : \beta = 0$ to establish a trend and the confidence interval can be inspected for inclusion of 1 to establish dose proportionality.

R produces the following output for weighted linear regression of log (Dose) on log (AUC):

```
Coefficients:
              Estimate Std. Error t value Pr(>|t|)
(Intercept)   -3.5042     1.9007   -1.844  0.13902
logAUC         2.2448     0.4451    5.044  0.00726 **
```

We indeed see that there is a significant trend. In addition, the CI for β does not include 1, which means that we cannot rule out dose proportionality. The R^2 for the regression is .83. We can plot the regression line with the confidence interval (shown in Figure 2.2) and/or the prediction interval using R package 'ggplot2':

```
>ggplot(new_df, aes(x=logDose, y=logAUC,weight = 1/ se.
hat^2,col="darkgrey"))+
  geom_point(size=5,col='grey')+
  geom_smooth(method=lm, se=TRUE,col='black')
```

Testing between doses or treatment groups can be implemented using contrasts as indicated above.

2.3 Related R Package 'PK'

Jaki and Wolfsegger [10] have provided noncompartmental PK analysis through the R package 'PK'. Estimation of various PK parameters, confidence intervals, and hypothesis testing is included in the package. Serial, complete, and incomplete designs and batch designs are considered in this useful package.

The following R code loads up the 'rats' data from Holder et al. [8] I analyzed earlier and produces the two-sided and one-sided confidence interval for dose 100 mg

```
> data(Rats)
> data <- subset(Rats,Rats$dose==100)
> # two-sided CI: data call
> auc(data=data,method=c('z','t'), design='batch')

Estimation for a batch design

              Estimate    SE      95% t-CI
AUC to tlast    39.47 7.31 (14.94;64.00)

              Estimate    SE      95% z-CI
AUC to tlast    39.47 7.31 (25.14;53.80)

> # one-sided CI: data call
> auc(data=data,method=c('z','t'), alternative="less", design=
'batch')
Estimation for a batch design

              Estimate    SE     95% t-CI
AUC to tlast    39.47 7.31 (21.60;Inf)

              Estimate    SE     95% z-CI
AUC to tlast    39.47 7.31 (27.45;Inf)
```

```
Comparing with the AUC for the 100 mg/kg dose from my previous
calculations:
```

```
> se.AUC.hat[1]
[1] 7.309978
```

Fortunately, the package has all the calculations already built-in for the ease of use of the statistician analyzing noncompartmental PK analysis.

3

Bioequivalence Studies

The World Health Organization (WHO) defines bioequivalence as 'two pharmaceutical products are bioequivalent if they are pharmaceutically equivalent or pharmaceutical alternatives, and their bioavailabilities, in terms of rate (Cmax and Tmax) and extent of absorption (AUC), after administration of the same molar dose under the same conditions, are similar to such a degree that their effects can be expected to be essentially the same' [28].

Bioequivalence is the study of two drugs for comparability (as stated above) of their bioavailability at the site of action. For example, two drugs with the same active ingredient may have different routes of administration and may need to be compared for bioequivalence. Another example is a drug, which may have changed its formulation during the drug development process and needs to be compared to the original formulation. In these cases, a bioequivalence study can be part of an NDA submission. PK parameters, like AUC, Cmax, and Tmax (time at which Cmax is achieved), are measured and analyzed for this purpose. The variables assume log normal distribution for analysis.

There are many designs of bioequivalence studies, such as the parallel design, multiarm parallel, replicate, crossovers, and others. The crossover design is an important basic flavor in these designs, where each patient received each of two (or more) drugs at different time points.

3.1 Crossover Equivalence Design and Composite Hypotheses

The order of receiving each treatment is randomized for the patient, denoted as *sequence*, the time points where they receive the treatment is denoted as *period*. In the simplest setting, we have two treatments (R for reference and T for test), two sequences (RR and TR), and two periods. This is known as the 2-2-2 bioequivalence study.

The TOST procedure (two one-sided tests) was developed to compare test and reference products for bioequivalence. Let μ_T and μ_R be the mean values of a PK parameter, and let the interval (θ_1, θ_2) be the interval of acceptance range for bioequivalence. FDA and other regulatory agencies have suggested to set $(\theta_1, \theta_2) = (0.8, 1.25)$ for most cases, although sometimes we do see wider (narrower) regions.

The composite bioequivalence hypotheses are based on the ratio μ_T/μ_R :

$$H_{0:}\ \mu_T/\mu_R \leq \theta_1 \text{ or } \mu_T/\mu_R \geq \theta_2 \text{ vs } H_1.\theta_1 < \mu_T/\mu_R < \theta_2$$

The hypothesis can also be formulated as the $\log\left(\mu_T/\mu_R\right)$.

3.1.1 R Code for Fitting Data from Crossover Design

In general, the model used to fit the data of a 2-2-2 study is a general linear model with factors Treatment, Sequence, Subject (Sequence), and Period.

$$\text{modA} = \text{lm}\left(\log\left(\text{AUC}\right) \sim \text{treatment} + \text{sequence}\right.$$
$$\left. + \text{subject} + \text{period, data} = \text{data}\right)$$

In addition, the linear mixed model of log-transformed PK response can also be used

$$\text{modB} = \text{lm}\left(\log\left(\text{CMAX}\right) \sim \text{treatment} + \text{sequence} + \text{period}\right.$$
$$\left. + \left(1\,|\,\text{subject}\right), \text{data} = \text{data}\right)$$

which can be evaluated with R lmerTest::lmer function

Bayesian models of analysis of the data are also prevalent. However, for the rest of the chapter we will assume the first model approach lm() for our discussions below.

Schutz, Labes, and Fuglsang [11] provide several useful data sets of varying degree of complexity in bioequivalence studies to compare parameter estimates and confidence intervals computed from R, SAS, WinNonlin, and so on. The objective was to demonstrate that R was yielding the same results as the other commercially available software on the market. All the data sets are downloadable from the journal's webpage.

The first few observations of a data set included in Schutz [11] look like the following:

```
> head(dta)
  ObsNumber Subj Trt Per Seq        Var
1         1    1   T   1  TR 168.40697
2         2    1   R   2  TR 210.91930
3         3    2   T   1  TR 131.03056
4         4    2   R   2  TR  67.43137
5         5    3   T   1  TR 151.73659
6         6    3   R   2  TR  85.12962
```

The variable could be AUC or Cmax, for example.
The linear model is fit using the R command

```
> lm(log(Var)~Trt+Per+Seq+Subj, data=dta)
```

The result of lm() is saved as an object called 'muddle' in the R code for Analyse222BE() function. The coefficient 'TrtT' is the difference T-R as 'TrtR' is set to zero. The direct estimate of ln(Test)/ln(Ref) is then the estimated coefficient for 'TrtT'. The 90% confidence interval can be estimated by using the confint() function on the muddle object for the 'TrtT' coefficient (R code: `confint(muddle,c("TrtT"), level=1-2*alpha)`, where alpha=.05).

The code is also downloadable from the journal website [11].

The output of anova() on the returned object of the model above returns the following:

```
Analysis of Variance Table

Response: log(Var)
              Df  Sum Sq Mean Sq  F value   Pr(>F)
Trt            1     2.0    2.02   2.9514  0.08624
Per            1   182.7  182.67 266.3575  < 2e-16
Seq            1   493.3  493.25 719.2209  < 2e-16
Subj         715  8095.4   11.32  16.5092  < 2e-16
Residuals    715   490.4    0.69
```

where the MSE is 0.69. This is important because the confidence interval of the log of the two means is $\log\left(\frac{A}{B}\right) \pm t-value * \sqrt{MSE*\left(\frac{1}{N_1}+\frac{1}{N_2}\right)}$.

This should give same result to the one obtained from confint() above by using the correct t-value for alpha=.05, MSE=.69 and N1 and N2 are # of subjects in sequence RT and TR. In balanced designs the same sizes are the same.

Also, often the coefficient for intraindividual variation is needed for computations and is defined by $CV_{intra}\% = 100\sqrt{e^{MSE}-1}$.

The script included in the Schutz paper [11] reports it as well:

```
Type III sum of squares: (mimicing SAS/SPSS but with Seq
tested against Subj)

log(Var)  ~  Trt + Per + Seq + Subj
              Df  Sum Sq Mean Sq   F value       Pr(>F)
Trt            1    1.60   1.595   2.32578      0.12769
Per            1  182.67 182.671 266.35748  < 2.22e-16
Seq            1  493.25 493.250  43.56485   7.9919e-11
Subj         715 8095.38  11.322  16.50920  < 2.22e-16
Residuals    715  490.36   0.686
```

```
Back-transformed PE and  90% confidence interval
CV (%) ...................................: 99.27
Point estimate (GMR).(%)..................: 93.42
Lower confidence limit.(%)...............: 86.81
Upper confidence limit.(%)...............: 100.55
```

As mentioned before, the FDA has recommended a range of 80%–125% for the 90% CI of the ratio of the product averages as the standard equivalence criterion. We see that the lower and upper limits reported above fall within the recommended range. Hence, the null hypothesis nonequivalence (H0: not equivalent) can be rejected.

3.2 Relevant R Packages

The design of bioequivalence studies is a vast topic and there are numerous R packages to analyze the data. As a sample of the packages, I want to mention two R packages that may help the statistician in conducting basic analysis of these experiments.

Above we show that the TOST procedure involves a composite hypotheses test. The procedure has been implemented in the R package 'PowerTOST' [12] for example. Power and sample size and confidence interval calculations are automated for a variety of bioequivalence designs including, parallel, crossover, crossover replicate, partial replicates, repeated crossovers, paired means, and others.

3.3 R Package 'BE'

The R package 'BE' [13] provides some very useful calculations for the 2 × 2 crossover design of bioequivalence. In case of this design, instead of the script I mentioned above from the Schutz paper [11], you could use this package in R. In this package, the example data set 'NCAResult4BE' is used several times to illustrate various functions. Note, AUC$_{0\text{-last}}$ calculates the AUC from time 0 to the last value above the limit of quantification.

```
>  head(NCAResult4BE)
   SUBJ GRP PRD TRT   AUClast    Cmax Tmax
1     1  RT   1   R 5018.927 1043.13 1.04
2     1  RT   2   T 6737.507  894.21 1.03
3     2  TR   1   T 4373.970  447.26 1.01
4     2  TR   2   R 6164.276  783.92 1.98
5     4  TR   1   T 5592.993  824.42 1.97
6     4  TR   2   R 5958.160  646.31 0.97
```

Some of the functions in this package include

- Analysis of bioequivalence test of a 2 × 2 study where the data are in similar format as above
- MSE calculation from confidence interval of previous 2 × 2 study
- CV calculation from MSE
- Plotting results of 2 × 2 study data
- Power using 2 × 2 previous study MSE
- Power using CV
- Sample Size

Simply using the following two commands, one is able to extract the following output and plots:

R commands

```
> write.csv(NCAResult4BE, "temp.csv", quote=FALSE, row.
names=FALSE)
> print(be2x2("temp.csv", c("AUClast")), na.print="")
```

R output

```
$AUClast
$AUClast$`Analysis of Variance (log scale)`
                 SS DF           MS           F          p
SUBJECT 2.875497e+00 32 8.985928e-02 3.183942248 0.0008742828
GROUP   1.024607e-01  1 1.024607e-01 1.145416548 0.2927731856
SUBJECT
(GROUP) 2.773036e+00 31 8.945279e-02 3.169539016 0.0009544080
PERIOD  3.027399e-05  1 3.027399e-05 0.001072684 0.9740824428
DRUG    3.643467e-02  1 3.643467e-02 1.290972690 0.2645764201
ERROR   8.749021e-01 31 2.822265e-02
TOTAL   3.786834e+00 65


$AUClast$`Between and Within Subject Variability`
                             Between Subject Within Subject
Variance Estimate                  0.03061507     0.02822265
Coefficient of Variation, CV(%)    17.63193968    16.91883011


$AUClast$`Least Square Means (geometric mean)`
                Reference Drug Test Drug
Geometric Means       5092.098  4858.245
```

```
$AUClast$`90% Confidence Interval of Geometric Mean
Ratio (T/R)`
                    Lower Limit Point Estimate Upper Limit
90% CI for Ratio       0.889436       0.9540753    1.023412

$AUClast$`Sample Size`
                        True Ratio=1 True Ratio=Point Estimate
80% Power Sample Size             6                          7
```

R plots

Figure 3.1 shows the boxplots of AUClast by sequence, period, and treatment. Figure 3.2 shows the spaghetti (individual plots) of the AUClast data. The solid and dashed lines separate the two groups with respect to their crossover treatment assignment.

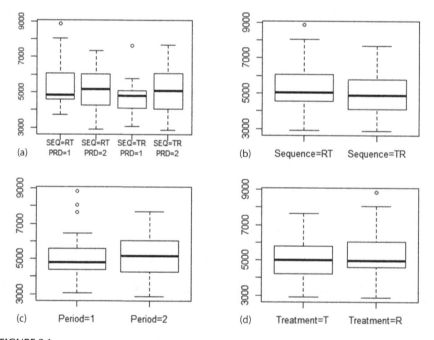

FIGURE 3.1
Box plots for AUClast. (a) By sequence and period, (b) by sequence, (c) by period, and (d) by treatment.

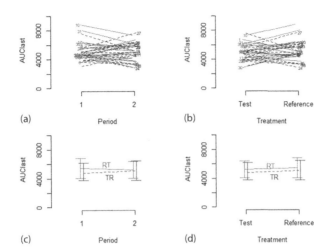

FIGURE 3.2
Equivalence plots for AUClast. (a) Individual plot for period, (b) individual plot for treatment, (c) mean and SD by period, and (d) mean and SD by treatment.

This chapter is intended to provide you with examples of doing R analysis of bioequivalence crossover study, which produces equivalent estimates to SAS and other commercially available software. Remember the endpoints are PK parameters of one or more biomarkers. There are numerous R packages and code scripts available for design and analysis of various types of bioequivalence designs. Once the reader is familiar with the basic design and analysis, custom code for more complex designs can be more readily created in R as needed.

4

Cross-Sectional Profile of Pharmacodynamics Biomarkers

Pharmacodynamic (PD) biomarkers need to be explored both longitudinally as well as for a particular time point (landmark analysis) for treatment effect. Usually, the marker is measured both at the start of the subject's participation in clinical trial and at least at one time point after commencing treatment. The biomarkers could be tissue or blood-based (serum or plasma), or from cerebrospinal fluid, urine, or any other biological samples collected from the patient. The assay could be uniplex or multiplex, resulting in a panel of biomarkers. Whether the disease area is cancer, cardiovascular, infectious, Alzheimer's, dental, or others, biomarkers play an increasingly significant role of clinical trial in developing precision medicine. The biomarkers help study the pharmacodynamic (PD) effect of the drug and are often a cheaper, less invasive way to monitor the disease outcome under study than the clinical endpoints(s). The biomarkers are not only studied by themselves under treatment and over time, but also their correlation with the end clinical outcome is often reported as building confidence for the biological mechanism of the drug on the disease.

4.1 Visualization and ANOVA

'A picture is worth a thousand words' is an adage that applies heavily in the analysis of PD effects of the drug through biomarker. The rapid development of statistical methodology coupled with increasing computing power has paved the way to provide visual summaries of multiplexed data.

The purpose of this chapter is to introduce a few basic visualization tools in this context. Assuming we are interested in the time point t (e.g., t could be 1 year of treatment), the common metrics plotted with biomarkers are as follows:

- Actual values at t = 1 year after treatment
- Change from baseline at time = t
- Percent change from baseline at time = t
- Area under the curve (AUC) of values (or changes from baseline) over several measurements from baseline to time = t

The underlying assumption I am making is that the biomarker is a continuous variable with the Gaussian distribution. Often the biomarker is log-transformed or square root transformed when there is significant departure from normality.

The mean and SE (or SD or CI) are plotted by dose at time = t as the first step of visualization. Here, is a sample data set and R code:

```
> head(pd)
          pd trt
1  15.216102   1
2  10.514347   1
3 -26.712865   1
4 -18.779960   1
5  31.062970   1
6  -2.795155   1
```

The pd data set contains percent change baseline at t=4 of PD's biomarker 'pd' weeks for multiple treatment (dose) levels with a drug. à The 'pd' data set contains percent change from baseline at t=4 months of PD biomarker data for several subjects. The variable 'trt' shows multiple treatment (dose) levels of the drug given to the different subjects.

A single, one line call to the function 'ggline' in the library 'ggpubr' will draw a nice plot of means and either standard deviation (SD), standard error (SE), or confidence interval (CI).

4.1.1 Mean and Standard Errors

```
>ggline(pd, x = "trt", y = "pd", legend.cex=.8,
        add = c("mean_se", "jitter"),
        title="Percent Change from Baseline at time=t\
        nbyTreatment\nmea n +/- SE",
        ylab = "PD Biomarker", xlab = "Treatment")
```

In Figure 4.1, one can see the dose levels are represented on the x-axis. Since placebo is designated as Treatment = 1, we can see that treatment dose group where Treatment = 3 has the biggest drop in percent change at time = t from starting treatment at t = 0.

For performing statistical tests for inference, I use the parametric ANOVA test and the nonparametric Kruskal–Wallis test to investigate whether the means (or medians) are the same as those in the treatment group. The following R code will implement the tests for making statistical inference:

```
>aov(pd~trt,data=pd)->res
>summary(res)
>pairwise.t.test(pd$pd,pd$trt,p.adjust.method = "BH")
>kruskal.test(pd$pd~pd$trt)
```

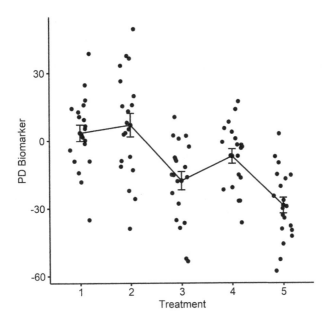

FIGURE 4.1
Lines connecting means and SE of biomarkers by treatment groups. The raw data is depicted as points.

First, the pairwise tests of equal means returns the Benjamini–Hochberg (BH) [16] corrected P values.

```
   1         2         3         4
2 0.53930  -         -         -
3 0.00055  9.6e-05   -         -
4 0.07276  0.02486   0.07276   -
5 5.8e-07  7.3e-08   0.07276   0.00050
```

Second, the Kruskal–Wallis rank–sum test of equal medians returns test statistics and P value.

```
        Kruskal-Wallis rank sum test

data:  pd$pd by pd$trt
Kruskal-Wallis chi-squared = 37.091, df = 4,
p-value = 1.725e-07
```

Both the pairwise test and the overall test show that treatment mean percent change from baselines is indeed different. A detailed description with examples of how to do ANOVA analysis in R is given in detail in the Statistical Tools for High Throughput Data Analysis website [15].

Violin plots and boxplots are popular visualization tools of the distribution of the data. Violin plots include the kernel density plot (rotated) on each side showing the shape of the distribution. Other related visualization code based on the R package 'ggplot2' are described in detail in the Statistical Tools for High Throughput Data Analysis website [14].

4.2 Violin Plots

The following R code generates the violin plots with the mean in the center for each dose group (Figure 4.2):

```
>p <- ggplot(pd, aes(x=trt, y=pd)) +
  labs(title=ttl,x="Dose Groups", y = "% change
  in PD biomarker")+ geom_violin(trim=FALSE, fill='#A4A4A4')
# violin plot with mean points
p + stat_summary(fun.y=mean, geom="point",shape=23, size=2)
```

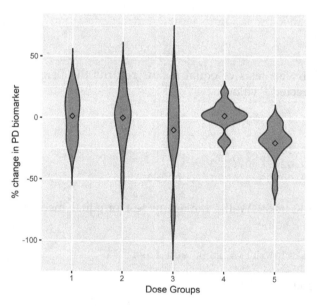

FIGURE 4.2
Violin plots of mean and SE of biomarker by dose groups.

If I want to add the boxplot as well to the plot, I use the following code:

```
>p <- ggplot(pd, aes(x=trt, y=pd)) +
   labs(title=ttl,x="Dose Groups", y = "% change in PD
   biomarker")+ geom_violin(trim=FALSE, fill='#A4A4A4')
   p+geom_boxplot(width=0.1, fill="white")
```

The output is given below (Figure 4.3):

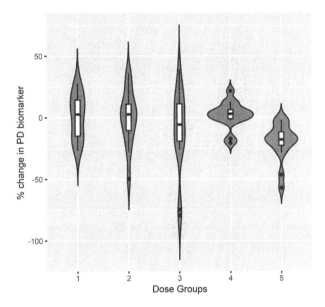

FIGURE 4.3
Violin + box plots of mean and SE of biomarker by dose groups.

The distribution of the percent change of the biomarker at time = t is shown for each dose level in the violins.

5

Timecourse Profile of Pharmacodynamics Biomarkers

Longitudinal profiles of pharmacodynamic (PD) biomarkers are studied for a variety of objectives. Showing a dose and time dependent trajectory of the biomarker is useful, but the marker could be further downstream from the mechanism of action. Nonetheless, through the analysis of these biomarkers, we provide supportive evidence for the drug action and/or disease modification. Pharmacodynamic biomarkers usually provide further understanding of the mechanistic pathway(s) between the drug and its impact on the disease. The objectives for the study of these biomarkers may yield early proof of concept (PoC), provide an early or alternate measurement of clinical response or even help clarify the safety profile. As an example, one could imagine the movement of a set of biomarkers indicating hepatic dysfunction in a subject.

In this chapter, we will be considering a single biomarker, but the analyses could be applied to multiple biomarkers. In most therapeutic areas, clinical trial measures more than one biomarker measured over time to monitor the disease. Looking at more than one PD biomarker will be covered later in Chapter 6 of this part of the book.

5.1 Visualization and Linear Mixed-Effects Model with Repeated Measures

Often biomarkers measured in the clinical trial are continuous, and the measurements follow an approximately normal distribution. As mentioned before, the log transformation and other boxcox transformation are available to apply to the data as needed. The linear mixed-effects model (MMRM) with repeated measures is used to examine the data, plot the model derived mean and confidence interval, and to make valid statistical inference on treatment effect over time or dose by time interaction.

Let us inspect the first few rows of our longitudinal data of our PD bio-marker 'pd' (long format) yields:

```
> head(pdlong)
          pd      base trt    time SUBJID
1 11.217347 18.65334   1 Month 1    S_1
2 -1.836234 19.95927   1 Month 1    S_2
3 35.262873 24.82207   1 Month 1    S_3
4 12.626589 25.17457   1 Month 1    S_4
5  9.475766 12.65688   1 Month 1    S_5
6  4.865109 15.66428   1 Month 1    S_6
```

The mixed-effects model was used to generate the means and CIs plotted below for treatment groups '1' (control) and '5' (highest dose) (Figure 5.1).

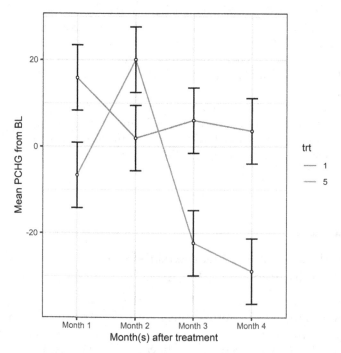

FIGURE 5.1
Mean and CI of PD biomarker by treatment group.

5.1.1 R Code for Plotting Percent Change from Baseline

The code to use to generate the above plot is:

```
>L=lmer(pd~base+trt*time+(1|SUBJID),data=pdlong[pdlong$trt
%in% c('1','5'),],REML=FALSE)
>d=summary(lsmeans(L,~trt*time))
```

The REML option is to set FALSE because we are interested in estimating the fixed effects.

```
>print(ggplot(d, aes(time)) +
        geom_line(aes(y = lsmean, group = trt,col=trt)) +
        geom_errorbar(aes(ymin = lower.CL, ymax = upper.CL),
        width = 0.2) +
        geom_point(aes(y = lsmean), size = 1, shape = 21,
        fill = "white") +
        labs(x = "Month(s) after treatment",
        y = "Mean PCHG from BL", title = paste("Mean Percent
            Change Over time\n","PD bioma rker",sep="")) +
        theme(plot.title=element_text(size=14))+
        theme_bw())
```

5.2 Time Varying Biomarker and Time-to-Event Outcome

The basic Cox proportional hazards model is defined as:

$$l(t|\mathbf{Z}) = l_0(t)\exp(\beta'Z)$$

where β is the covariate coefficient vector and $l_0(t)$ is the baseline hazard function over time. The hazard ratio $\exp(\beta'Z)$ depends on the covariates (like, age, sex, treatment, etc.) but not on time. When a patient biomarker(s) vary over time, we need mechanisms other than the time-independent covariate (usually baseline variables) adjustment model.

The Cox proportional hazards model with time varying covariate is defined as:

$$l(t|\mathbf{Z}) = l_0(t)\exp\left[\beta'Z(t)\right]$$

This model shows that the hazard at time t depends on the covariates at time t, Z(t). Now, the interpretation of parameter estimates has changed, but we still call this model proportional hazards model in a loose sense.

- In the time-independent setting, the model compares the survival distribution over time between covariate status (e.g., positive vs negative)
- In the time-dependent setting, the model compares the risk of event at each event time t between covariate status at that time of subjects in the risk set at time t

The partial likelihood mechanism is still used to evaluate the parameters and obtain MLE estimates. The partial likelihood is the conditional probability of choosing individual i to fail from the risk set, given the risk set at time X_i and given that one failure is to occur [17].

5.2.1 R Code for Modeling Time-Dependent Covariates in Survival Analysis

Therneau et al. [18], in R package 'survival', have incorporated continuous time-dependent coefficients $\beta(t)$ through the ordinary Cox model mechanism. The authors point out that the ordinary coxph function can be fooled to fit the time-dependent covariate data. The trick is to code time-dependent covariates using intervals of time.

Let us examine the data set 'scr' from the clinical study to investigate the chronic renal allograft dysfunction in renal transplants contained in the R 'mdhglm' package [19]. The renal function was evaluated from the serum creatinine (sCr) values. The event, which is a single terminating survival time (graft-loss time) measured in months, is observed from each patient. During the study period, there were 13 graft losses due to the kidney dysfunction. The data set contained 1395 observations with 9 variables. I added the 'start' time to the data set to be able to use the R 'coxph' function.

The following R code shows the first few lines of the data set:

```
>library(mdhglm)
>data(scr)

>tmp=NULL
>sid=unique(scr$id)
>for (i in 1:length(sid)) {
D=scr[scr$id==sid[i],]
l=nrow(D)
tmp=c(tmp,c(0,D$month[1:l-1]))
}
```

```
>scr$start=tmp
> head(scr)
       id    month   cr sex age       icr sur_time status first   start
1 7804 47.6066 1.6   1  34 0.6250000  57.4098       0     1  0.0000
2 7804 50.4918 1.3   1  34 0.7692308  57.4098       0     0 47.6066
3 7804 54.0656 1.6   1  34 0.6250000  57.4098       0     0 50.4918
4 7804 57.4098 1.2   1  34 0.8333333  57.4098       0     0 54.0656
5 7908 42.2295 0.9   1  48 1.1111111  59.8033       0     1  0.0000
6 7908 47.9344 1.3   1  48 0.7692308  59.8033       0     0 42.2295
```

Above we see that subject 7804 had creatinine levels of 1.6, 1.3, 1.6, and 1.2 at time intervals (0, 47.6066], (47.6066, 50.4918], (50.4918, 54.0656], and (54.0656, 57.4098], respectively. The last row for the subject shows the event status in the variable 'status'. The start and stop (=month) variables are necessary to invoke coxph(). A few caveats about setting up this type of data set are as follows: (i) the time-varying covariate cannot look forward in time, that is, cannot include observations beyond the event time, (ii) that data needs to be measured between baseline and event/censor time, (iii) that subjects cannot have multiple events, and (iv) that subjects cannot appear in overlapping intervals. If the data fall into these exceptions, then other methods to analyze the data must be considered.

Following is the R code to model time to the event = graft-loss with age as a time invariant variable, and creatinine as the time-varying covariate:

```
> fit=coxph(Surv(start,month,status)~age+cr,data=scr)
> fit
Call:
coxph(formula = Surv(start, month, status)
~ age + cr, data = scr)

        coef exp(coef)  se(coef)      z       p
age -0.0275    0.9728    0.0109  -2.52   0.012
cr   0.5450    1.7246    0.0361  15.08  <2e-16

Likelihood ratio test=209   on 2 df, p=0
n= 1395, number of events= 134
```

We can see that creatinine, a time-varying covariate, is significantly associated with time to graft loss. There is a 72.46% increase in the expected hazard relative to a one-point increase in creatinine keeping the age constant.

5.3 Comparing Three Ways of Modeling Longitudinal Biomarkers and a Time-to-Event Outcome

There is a lot of interest now in joint modeling of primary endpoint of the trial (e.g., binary response or time-to-event analysis on death, progression, or another event) and the longitudinally collected biomarker data. Numerous statistical methodologies have been proposed in the statistical literature to study the joint model in frequentist and Bayesian paradigms. In this section, I will address the joint modeling of time-to-event outcomes from patients and longitudinal biomarkers in the frequentist paradigm of maximum likelihood estimation.

There are three approaches to model the clinical outcome and the longitudinally collected biomarker data:

1. Separate analysis: Separate analyses of the biomarker data with linear mixed-effects model and the survival data with Cox proportional hazards model are carried out routinely. The limitation of this approach is that the biomarker data may be impacted by *informative censoring*, whereby the more severely diseased patients will have fewer biomarker measurements. This phenomenon cannot be addressed unless a common process accounts for the co-occurrence of the biomarker data and the clinical outcome.

2. Time dependent covariate: Time dependent covariate in survival analysis has been introduced above and is a commonly used procedure where the biomarker changes values over time and can be accommodated in the survival model. However, this model is best for *exogenous* time-dependent covariates – not endogenous biomarker data. The exogenous covariates, for example transplant status, can be modeled with time intervals and not assumed to be changing in between visits. However, biomarker data will have random variation and only assessed at schedule visit dates.

3. Joint modeling: Rizopoulous [25] has provided the statistical framework for joint modeling of the processes (biomarker and survival data) through maximum likelihood estimation whereby the biomarker can be assumed to have measurement error. The joint modeling framework assumes two submodels which share common parameters which is shown below.

Let T_i and C_i be respectively the potential failure and censoring times for patient i in the study. Let $\delta_i = I(T_i < C_i)$ be a survival status indicator and $U_i = \min(T_i, C_i)$ the observed failure or censoring time, whichever occurs first.

Let $z_i = 1$ be the treatment indicator taking value 0 or 1 if patient i is assigned to a control or a new treatment group;

In addition, $y_i(t)$ is a continuous biomarker variable collected longitudinally over time t with measurement error.

The individual patient i survival function is:

$$S_i(t|M_i(t)) = e^{\left\{-\int_0^t h_i(s|M_i(s))ds\right\}}$$

where $M_i(t) = \{m_i(s), 0 \leq s < t\}$ denotes the history of the true and unobserved values of the longitudinal process up to time t. We see that the survival function depends on the whole biomarker trajectory over time t.

5.3.1 R Package JM

R package JM [26] implements this joint model in R for survival and continuous biomarker. The first-order model is given by

$$h_i(t \mid M_i(t)) = h_0(t)e^{\left\{\gamma'x_i + \alpha_0 m_i(t) + \alpha_1 m_i'(t)\right\}}$$

where α_1 is the coefficients of the derivative or slope of $m_i(t)$; α_0 is the coefficient or intercept of $m_i(t)$ and γ is the coefficient of the baseline covariates

$$y_i(t) = m_i(t) + \varepsilon_i(t),$$

where $y_i(t)$ is the observed biomarker values at time t – and the $m_i(t)$ is the shared parameter which can be expanded into fixed and random effects.

Thus we see that the two sub-models (cox proportional hazards model and mixed effects model) framework is used simultaneously to estimate the model parameters.

5.3.2 Analysis of the AIDS Data Set

The AIDS data set is used in the JM package [26] which consists of 467 patients with AIDS virus who were treated with antiretroviral drugs and who had previously failed or were intolerant to zidovudine therapy. The objective of the study was to compare the efficacy and safety of two alternative antiretroviral drugs, namely didanosine (ddI) and zalcitabine (ddC) in the time-to-death. Patients were randomized to receive either ddI or ddC, and CD4 cell counts were recorded at study entry, as well as at 1, 6, 12, and 18 months.

5.3.2.1 R Code

```
library(mdhglm); library(lme4); library(survival);libra
ry(nlme);library(JM)

data("aids")
head(aids)
aids$gender = factor(aids$gender, levels =
c("male", "female"))
aids$drug = factor(aids$drug, levels = c("ddC", "ddI"))
aids$obstime = as.numeric(as.character(aids$obstime))

is.unsorted(aids$patient)
length(unique(aids$patient))
##  make newid that is unsorted
no.rows <- rle(c(aids$patient))
aids$newid <- paste0(rep( rep(LETTERS, length.out=467), no.
rows$lengths), aids$patient)
is.unsorted(aids$newid)
length(unique(aids$newid))

aids.id <- aids[!duplicated(aids$patient),]

# Model 1: Longitudinal model
lmeFit.aids <- lme(CD4~obstime + gender + obstime:drug,
random=~obstime|newid, data=aids)
sum=round(summary(lmeFit.aids)$tTable[,c(1, 2, 5)], 3)
int=round(intervals(lmeFit.aids)[[1]][, c(1,3)], 3)
lm.out = data.frame(sum[, 1],
                    paste("(", int[,1], ", ", int[,2], ")"),
                    sum[,2:3])
colnames(lm.out)=c("Estimate", "95% CI", "SE", "P")
lm.out$P = ifelse(lm.out$P==0.000, "<0.001", lm.out$P)
row.names(lm.out)=c("Intercept", "obstime", "genderfemale",
"obstime:drugddI")


# Model 2: Cox model
tdep.rrt <- coxph(Surv(start, stop, death) ~ drug
+ gender + CD4, data = aids)
hrci1=round(summary(tdep.rrt)$conf.int[, -2], 3) # HR and its CI
est1=round(summary(tdep.rrt)$coefficients[, c(1, 3, 5)], 3) #
coefficients, SE, and P
eci1=round(confint(tdep.rrt), 3) # estimates' CI
cox.out1=data.frame(est1[, 1],
                    paste("(",eci1[,1], eci1[,2], ")"),
                    est1[,2:3],
```

```
                          hrci1[,1],
                          paste("(",hrci1[,2], hrci1[,3], ")"))
cox.out1$P=ifelse(cox.out1$P==0, "<0.001", cox.out1$P)
colnames(cox.out1)=c("Estimate", "95% CI", "SE", "P", "HR",
"HR_95%CI")

## Model 3: Joint model

# Cox sub-model
coxFit.aids <- coxph(Surv(Time,death)~drug + gender +
CD4,data=aids.id, x=TRUE)

jointFit.aids <- jointModel(lmeFit.aids, coxFit.aids, timeVar=
"obstime",method="piecewise-PH-aGH")
sum.joint=summary(jointFit.aids)
attributes(sum.joint)

sum.long=summary(jointFit.aids)[[1]][,c(1, 2, 4)]
out.long = data.frame(round(sum.long[,1], 3),
                paste("( ", round(sum.long[,1]-1.96*sum.
                long[,2], 3), round(sum.long[,1]+1.96*sum.
                long[,2], 3), ")"),
                round(sum.long[,2], 3), ifelse(round(sum.
                long[,3], 3)==0.000, "< 0.001", round(sum.
                long[,3], 3)))
colnames(out.long) = c("Estimate", "95%CI", "SE", "P")
write.csv(out.long, "Table4.1_Jioint.MMRM_estimates_CI_p.
csv", row.names=T)

sum.cox=summary(jointFit.aids)[[2]][,c(1, 2, 4)]
ll = sum.cox[,1]-1.96*sum.cox[,2]
ul = sum.cox[,1]+1.96*sum.cox[,2]
out.cox = data.frame(Estimate=round(sum.cox[,1], 3),
                CI=paste("( ", round(ll, 3),
                round(ul, 3), ")"),
                SE=round(sum.cox[,2], 3),
                P=ifelse(round(sum.cox[,3], 3)==0.000,
                "< 0.001", round(sum.cox[,3], 3)),
                HR = round(exp(sum.cox[,1]),3),
                HR95ci = paste("(", round(exp(ll), 3),
                round(exp(ul), 3), ")"))
colnames(out.cox) = c("Estimate", "95%CI", "SE", "P", "HR",
"HR_95%CI")
```

5.3.2.2 Results

1. The separate analysis approach yielded the following results
(Table 5.1):

TABLE 5.1

AIDS Data – Results of Separate Analyses on Endpoint

	Estimate	95% CI	SE
Intercept	7.116	(6.658, 7.573)	0.233
Obstime	−0.163	(−0.204, −0.122)	0.021
Genderfemale	0.764	(−0.689, 2.218)	0.74
obstime:drugddI	0.028	(−0.03, 0.087)	0.03

In the interaction term above, we see there does not seem to be a differential effect on the average longitudinal evolution of CD4 (biomarker) in the two treatment group of patients in the trial.

2. The cox proportional hazards model with time dependent covariate yielded (Table 5.2):

TABLE 5.2

AIDS Data – Results of Analyzing Time Dependent Covariate in Cox Proportional Hazards Model

	Estimate	95% CI	SE	P	HR	HR_95%CI
drugddI	0.185	(−0.009, 0.378)	0.099	0.061	1.203	(0.991, 1.46)
genderfemale	−0.02	(−0.377, 0.336)	0.182	0.91	0.98	(0.686, 1.399)
CD4	−0.158	(−0.187, −0.13)	0.015	<0.001	0.854	(0.83, 0.878)

The effect of CD4 on log HR is −0.158 (SE = 0.015) and this is different from the joint model result below. The treatment effect is not significant.

3. In the joint model code above, note that the option='piecewise-PH-GH' indicates a proportional hazards model with piecewise-constant baseline hazard. And the 'GH' indicated the gauss hermite integration rule applied to the integral of the joint log likelihood of the shared parameter sub-models [25].

The joint model yielded (Table 5.3):

TABLE 5.3

AIDS Data – Results of Joint Modeling – Longitudinal Endpoint

	Estimate	95% CI	SE	P
(Intercept)	6.919	(6.497, 7.342)	0.216	<0.001
obstime	−0.095	(−0.173, −0.017)	0.04	0.017
genderfemale	1.778	(0.646, 2.91)	0.578	0.002
obstime:drugddI	0.066	(−0.028, 0.161)	0.048	0.17

The treatment effect is not significant (Table 5.4).

TABLE 5.4

AIDS Data – Results of Joint Modeling – Survival Endpoint

	Estimate	95% CI	SE	P	HR	HR_95%CI
drugddI	0.256	(−0.034, 0.545)	0.148	0.083	1.292	(0.967, 1.725)
genderfemale	0.191	(−0.292, 0.674)	0.247	0.439	1.21	(0.746, 1.963)
CD4	−0.182	(−0.225, −0.138)	0.022	<0.001	0.834	(0.799, 0.871)
Assoct	0.01	(−0.039, 0.059)	0.025	0.685	1.01	(0.962, 1.061)
log(xi.1)	−2.919	(−3.382, −2.456)	0.236	<0.001	0.054	(0.034, 0.086)
log(xi.2)	−2.407	(−2.865, −1.949)	0.234	<0.001	0.09	(0.057, 0.142)
log(xi.3)	−1.975	(−2.533, −1.417)	0.285	<0.001	0.139	(0.079, 0.242)
log(xi.4)	−2.453	(−3.183, −1.723)	0.373	<0.001	0.086	(0.041, 0.179)
log(xi.5)	−2.285	(−2.968, −1.602)	0.349	<0.001	0.102	(0.051, 0.202)
log(xi.6)	−2.233	(−3.072, −1.394)	0.428	<0.001	0.107	(0.046, 0.248)
log(xi.7)	−2.105	(−3.157, −1.054)	0.537	<0.001	0.122	(0.043, 0.349)

The effect of CD4 on log HR is −0.182 (SE = 0.022) and this different from the cox proportional hazards model with time dependent covariate result above.

5.4 Forest Plots for Linking Changes in Outcome to Changes in a Single PD Marker

Forest plots are used in meta-analysis and are available via several R packages. It is a popular and powerful way of seeing the change in a statistical parameter (for example, hazard ratio of the outcome of interest) by different biomarker subgroups. For a single PD biomarker – for example, we may categorize the change from baseline at time $t = 6$ months, into quartiles in the following way:

- Percent change in biomarker value from baseline > 0
  - The biomarker of interest did not decrease but stayed the same or increased at time t relative to baseline
- Percent change in biomarker value from baseline decreased up to 10% from baseline
- Percent change in biomarker value from baseline decreased between 10% and 20% from baseline
- Percent change in biomarker value from baseline decreased more than 20% from baseline

The forest plot below shows this categorization: we expect to see mostly placebo subjects in the first category and mostly treated subjects in the category where the biomarker has been modulated downwards the most. We can see that in subjects with decreasing levels of change in biomarker at time = t – receive increasing treatment benefit.

5.4.1 R Code

First, the R code, followed by the output (Figure 5.2):

```
library(forestplot)
test_data <- data.frame(coef=c(2.45, 1.4,.9,0.43),
                        low=c(1.5, 1.1, .7,0.25),
                        high=c(4, 3, 1.7, 0.75),
                        boxsize=c(0.2,0.2,0.2,0.2))
row_names <- cbind(c("Biomarker",
                "Biomarker %change>0",
```

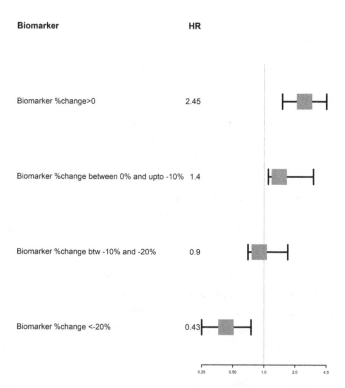

FIGURE 5.2
Hazard ratio of onset of dementia vs biomarker %change at time = t.

```
                         "Biomarker %change between 0%
                         and upto -10%",
                         "Biomarker %change btw -10% and -20%",
                         "Biomarker %change <-20%"),c("HR", test_
data$coef))
test_data <- rbind(rep(NA, 5), test_data)
forestplot(labeltext = row_names,
           title=paste("Hazard Ratio of Onset
of Dementia\n vs Biomarker %Change at time=t"),
           test_data[,c("coef", "low", "high")],
           is.summary=c(TRUE,FALSE, FALSE,FALSE,FALSE),
           boxsize = test_data$boxsize,
           zero = 1,
           xlog = TRUE,colgap=unit(.6,"mm"),
           lwd.ci=2, ci.vertices=TRUE, ci.vertices.
           height = 0.1,
           col = fpColors(lines="black", box="darkgrey"))
```

This example of categorizing change from baseline is drawn from a data set I am currently working on, but of course, you will choose a way of categorization that is meaningful to your work. You may simply look at two categories: increased vs decreased, or decreased by 1 SD, 2 SDs, and so on. The treatment shows statistically significant effect (beneficial) for the subgroup of subjects with more than 20% decline in the biomarker level since baseline visit.

6

Evaluating Multiple Biomarkers

6.1 Forest Plots for Linking Changes in Outcome to Changes in Multiple PD Marker

Forest plots can be used to compare treatment effects in clinical trial across several factors. In this section, we see the results of comparing treatment and placebo groups, simultaneously for several subgroups, with respect to hazard ratio as the clinical outcome. The subgroups considered for the example include (i) a clinical variable; (ii) a demographic variable; (iii) four biomarkers (marker 1 is simply categorized as positive or negative (baseline or at time t); marker 2 is categorized as percent change in baseline @t=6 months (as an example) having increased vs decreased; marker 3 change from baseline at time t has been categorized as less than or equal to a threshold (X) or greater; marker 4 has been categorized as percentage change less than 50% or more than or equal to 50%).

The data set and code were inspired from the R bloggers website [23]. The data are a data frame containing a toy example of fabricated data. The filename is forestplot.csv and is given in Table 6.1.

6.1.1 R Code

The R package 'forestplot' [24] is used to plot the graph. First is the section of the code that reads in the data:

```
datafile <- file.path("ForestPlotData.csv")
data <- read.csv(datafile, stringsAsFactors=FALSE)

## Labels defining subgroups are a little indented!
subgps <- c(4,5,8,9,12,13,16,17,20,21,24,25)
data$Variable[subgps] <- paste("  ",data$Variable[subgps])

## Combine the count and percent column
np <- ifelse(!is.na(data$Count), paste(data$Count,"
(",data$Percent,")",sep=""), NA)
## The rest of the columns in the table.
```

TABLE 6.1

Data summaries for Forest Plots

Variable	Count	Percent	Point Estimate	Low	High	Control Group	Treated Group	P Value
Overall	1000	100	0.8	0.5	1.1	30	18	
Clinical 1								0.05
<=median	650	65	1.5	1.05	1.9	22	23	
>median	350	35	0.8	0.6	1.25	22.1	18.2	
Demog 1								0.13
Cat 1	612	61	1.3	1.05	1.9	16.8	13.5	
Cat 2	388	39	0.7	0.5	1.1	18.3	22.9	
Biomarker 1								0.52
Positive	400	40	1.05	0.6	1.8	22.3	23.4	
Negative	600	60	1.2	0.6	1.6	18.3	17.9	
%Change in Biomarker 2 @6 mos								0.04
<=0%	450	45	0.56	0.44	0.8	32	16	
>0%	550	55	1.2	0.9	1.4	18	20	
Change in Biomarker 3 @6 mos								0.38
<=X	300	30	1.4	0.9	1.9	20.1	16.2	
>X	700	70	1.1	0.8	1.4	15.6	15.3	
%Change in Biomarker 4 @6 mos								0.033
<50%	700	70	1.2	0.8	1.5	22.6	20.4	
>=50%	300	30	0.66	0.5	0.8	20.7	11.1	

```
tabletext <- cbind(c("Subgroup","\n",data$Variable),
                c("No. of Patients (%)","\n",np),
                c("t-Yr Cum. Event Rate\n Placebo",
                   "\n",data$Control.Grp),
                c("t-Yr Cum. Event Rate\n Treated",
                   "\n",data$Treated.Grp),
                c("P Value","\n",data$P.Value))
```

Next the section which calls 'forestplot':

```
forestplot(labeltext=tabletext, graph.pos=3,
           mean=c(NA,NA,data$Point.Estimate),
           lower=c(NA,NA,data$Low), upper=c(NA,NA,data$High),
           title="Hazard Ratio",
           xlab="      <---Trt Better---    ---Pl Better--->",
           hrzl_lines=TRUE,
```

```
txt_gp=fpTxtGp(label=gpar(cex=.7),
               ticks=gpar(cex=1),
               xlab=gpar(cex = .8),
               title=gpar(cex = 1)),
graphwidth="auto",
col=fpColors(box="darkgrey", lines="black",
zero = "gray75"),
zero=1, cex=0.9, lineheight = "auto", boxsize=.3,
colgap=unit(.6,"mm"),
lwd.ci=2, ci.vertices=TRUE, ci.vertices.height = 0.4)
```

The output is shown in Figure 6.1.

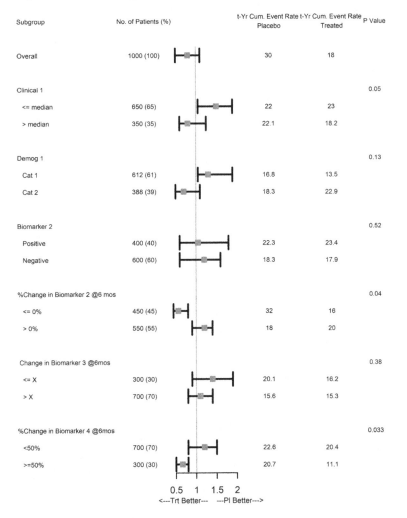

FIGURE 6.1
Hazard Ratio (treatment effect) by different subgroups.

Clearly, Percent changes in Biomarker 2 (with decreased levels) and Biomarker 4 (with more than 50% increase) are seen to have differential treatment benefits.

Similar plots can be easily made for odds ratio or regression slope parameters as the clinical outcomes.

6.2 Network Analysis

Network or graphs provide a very useful mathematical representation of complex biological systems or therapeutics effects on such systems. Although this topic will be covered in numerous parts of this book, this chapter is the introduction to the network analysis. Statistical summaries like correlations or P values can be represented as *edges* of the network graph and the *nodes* or *vertices* would be random variables. The whole network then would be a summary of the interconnectedness (strength, direction, type of relationship) among the variables. We are interested in estimating the topology of the true network, which is unknown, through statistical modeling.

In this chapter, we are concerned with introducing graphical model basic terminology and making visual representations of the graph. Even though it is possible to have directed graphs (perhaps pointing to causal relationships), we will focus on undirected graphs where the variables x and y are considered unordered. Choosing correlation as the initial metric for the edges, we can denote the magnitude by the thickness of the line and the type of association (positive vs negative) by the color of the line. A network of nodes and their interconnectedness is represented by an *adjacency matrix*. For the undirected network, we can assume that the adjacency matrix is symmetric.

When a set of biomarkers measure the activity rhythms of a biological organ or system or have a common basis for co-occurrence, then we can use network analysis to quantify the inter-relatedness in a multivariate fashion. We need not distinguish which are predictors and which are outcomes like in linear regression. We can include biomarkers and clinical variables (demographics, treatment) in the same model. Alternatively, we can model the network of biomarkers separately for each treatment group. We assume that the data set is contemporaneous in this analysis, for example, each biomarker variable could percentage change from baseline at time = t (days, weeks, months, or years). The network would show the pairwise correlations between the percentage changes in the biomarker variables.

The data set we will use to visualize a model of the inter-relatedness of biomarkers will be the estrogen gene data set [20]. First, we read in, normalize, and identify genes with significant effects. It is an Affymetrix microarray data set. There is no specific reason for choosing this data set. After reading in and normalizing the data using standard pre-processing tools in R, we chose 10 of the most significant upregulated and 10 of the most significant downregulated genes from the standard pipeline of identifying and ranking the genes. The variable 'estrogenMainEffects' contains numeric data of these 20 genes. We rename the genes to generic Biomarker 1, Biomarker 2, and so on to make the variable names more relevant to our interest.

Next, we create the adjacency matrix of a graph with the pairwise correlation of each of the biomarkers or genes. The R package 'igraph' [21] was installed and used to construct the graphical model of the vertices (genes) and adjacency (correlations) edges. This is very useful, except the limitation that correlations have been thought of producing spurious edges and not distinguishing between direct (causal or predictive) and indirect (associative) relationships. You can show partial correlations or Euclidean distance in place of correlations. That would produce a more parsimonious multivariate model. The term Gaussian graphical models is used to denote multivariate normal distribution and the corresponding variance–covariance matrix when the biomarker variables are continuous and approximately normally distributed. Conditional independence between the variables is represented in the graph by the absence of edges. The measure of conditional independence is achieved through partial correlations. More details on partial correlation networks are given in Section IV.

As mentioned above, the graph we build is undirected. The adjacency matrix is a square matrix p × p, where there are p biomarkers in the data set, for example. Of course, additional variables can be added, including but not limited to continuous variables, into the analysis. We will focus on the example of modeling the inter-relationships of p biomarkers in this example.

6.2.1 R Code

```
#To install, use
BiocManager::install(c("affy","estrogen","vsn","genefilter"))
library(affy)
library(estrogen)
library(vsn)
library(genefilter)
datadir <- system.file("extdata", package="estrogen")
dir(datadir)
setwd(datadir)
pd <- read.AnnotatedDataFrame("estrogen.txt", header=TRUE,
sep="", row.names=1)
a <- ReadAffy(filenames=rownames(pData(pd)), phenoData=pd,
verbose=TRUE)
# Normalise the data
x <- expresso(
a,
bgcorrect.method="rma",
normalize.method="constant",
```

```
pmcorrect.method="pmonly",
summary.method="avgdiff")
# Remove control probes
controlProbeIdx <- grep("^AFFX", rownames(x))
x <- x[-controlProbeIdx,]
# Identify genes of significant effect
lm.coef <- function(y) lm(y ~ estrogen * time.h)$coefficients
eff <- esApply(x, 1, lm.coef)
effectUp <- names(sort(eff[2,], decreasing=TRUE)[1:10])
effectDown <- names(sort(eff[2,], decreasing=FALSE)[1:10])
main.effects <- c(effectUp, effectDown)
# Filter the expression set object to include only genes of
significant effect
estrogenMainEffects <- exprs(x)[main.effects,]
head(estrogenMainEffects)

library(igraph)
library(ggplot2)

corMat=cor(t(estrogenMainEffects))
rownames(corMat)=colnames(corMat)=paste("BM",rep(1:length(V(g)
$name)),sep="_")

# Reorder the correlation matrix
cormat <- reorder_cormat(corMat)
corMat[corMat<.6]=0
upper_tri <- get_upper_tri(cormat)
# Melt the correlation matrix
melted_cormat <- melt(upper_tri, na.rm = TRUE)
g <- graph.adjacency(corMat,
mode="undirected",
weighted=TRUE,
diag=FALSE
)

# Colour negative correlation edges as grey
E(g)[which(E(g)$weight<0)]$color <- "grey"
# Colour positive correlation edges as black
E(g)[which(E(g)$weight>0)]$color <- "black"
# Convert edge weights to absolute values
E(g)$weight <- abs(E(g)$weight)
# Assign names to the graph vertices as biomarkers - do this
step only if you want to rename vars
V(g)$name <- paste("BM",rep(1:length(V(g)$name)),sep="_")
# Change shape of graph vertices
V(g)$color <- "lightgrey"
# Change colour of vertex frames
V(g)$vertex.frame.color <- "orange"
# Scale the size of the vertices to be proportional to the
level of expression of each gene represented by each vertex
```

```
# Multiply scaled vales by a factor of 10
scale01 <- function(x){(x-min(x))/(max(x)-min(x))}
vSizes <- (scale01(apply(estrogenMainEffects, 1, mean)) + 1.0)
* 10
# Amplify or decrease the width of the edges
edgeweights <- E(g)$weight * 2.0
# Plot the tree object
plot(
g,
layout=layout.fruchterman.reingold,
edge.curved=TRUE,
vertex.size=vSizes,
vertex.label.dist=-0.5,
vertex.label.color="black",
asp=FALSE,
vertex.label.cex=0.6,
edge.width=edgeweights,
edge.arrow.mode=0,
main="Network Correlation Graph"
)
```

6.2.2 Network Correlation Graph

Biomarker BM1 (e.g., percent change from baseline at time=t) seems to not be associated with changes in the other biomarkers, whereas there is a good agreement between percent changes in BM17, BM18, and BM20. I note that the same information could be visualized by a heatmap, although the interrelatedness information is not quite obvious (Figure 6.2).

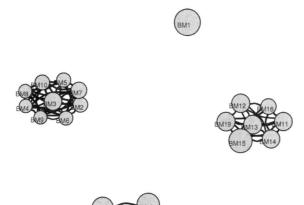

FIGURE 6.2
Network Correlation Graph for top biomarkers.

6.3 Visualization Through Heatmaps

The heatmap is provided here to corroborate the information of the network analysis.

We see the same clusters between the changes in the biomarkers as in the network analysis.

```
#Heatmap
colnames(melted_cormat)[1:2]=c("Biomarker1","Biomarker2")
# Create a ggheatmap
ggheatmap <- ggplot(melted_cormat, aes(Biomarker1, Biomarker2,
fill = value))+ geom_tile(color = "white")+
   scale_fill_gradient2(low = "black", high = "darkgrey",
                        mid = "white",
                        midpoint = 0, limit = c(-1,1), space =
                        "Lab",
                        name="Pearson\nCorrelation") +
                        theme_minimal()+ # minimal theme
   theme(axis.text.x = element_text(angle = 45, vjust = 1,
                        size = 12, hjust = 1))+ coord_fixed()
# Print the heatmap
print(ggheatmap+ggtitle("Correlation between top biomarkers"))
```

The heatmap below is a 2D visual representation of the upper triangular correlation matrix. The code is given above. Mode details about heatmaps in ggplot() is available in the documentation of the package [22] (Figure 6.3).

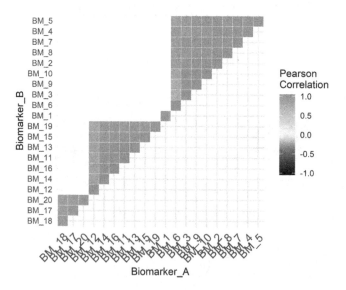

FIGURE 6.3
Heatmap showing Correlation between top biomarkers.

Note that in addition to using heatmap for correlation, we could also produce a heatmap for the percent change values of the biomarkers, with time t as rows and subjects' IDs as columns, followed by hierarchical clustering. This would show you if there are differential patterns of covariations between the two clusters. If there is, then the clusters may well align with the treatment group or a prognostic factor. We will discuss this type of heatmap in Section II of the book.

References

1. https://en.wikipedia.org/wiki/Biomarker_(medicine)
2. Morgan P, Van Der Graaf PH, Arrowsmith J, Feltner DE, Drummond KS, Wegner CD, Street SD. (2011). Can the flow of medicines be improved? Fundamental pharmacokinetic and pharmacological principles toward improving phase II survival. *Drug Discov. Today*, 17:419–424. doi:10.1016/j.drudis.2011.12.020.
3. Cartwright ME, Cohen S, Fleishaker JC, Madani S, Mcleod JF, Musser B, Williams SA. (2010). Proof of concept: A PhRMA position paper with recommendations for best practice. *Clin. Pharmacol. Ther.*, 87:278–285. doi:10.1038/clpt.2009.286.
4. Parchment RE, Doroshow JH. (2016). Pharmacodynamic endpoints as clinical trial objectives to answer important questions in oncology drug development. *Semin. Oncol.*, 43(4):514–525. doi:10.1053/j.seminoncol.2016.07.002
5. Bailer AJ. (1988). Testing for the equality of area under the curves when using destructive measurement techniques. *J. Pharmacokinet Biopharm.*, 16(3):303–309.
6. Nedelman JR, Gibiansky E, Lau DT. (1995). Applying Bailer's method for AUC confidence intervals to sparse sampling. *Pharm Res.*, 12(1):124–128.
7. Wolfsegger MJ, Jaki T. (2005). Estimation of AUC from 0 to infinity in serial sacrifice designs. *J. Pharmacokinet. Pharmacodyn.* 32:757. doi:10.1007/s10928-005-0044-0.
8. Holder DJ, Hsuan F, Dixit R, Soper K. (1999). A method for estimating and testing area under the curve in serial sacrifice, batch, and complete data designs. *J. Biopharm. Stat.*, 9(3):451–464. doi:10.1081/BIP-100101187.
9. https://stats.idre.ucla.edu/r/library/r-library-contrast-coding-systems-for-categorical-variables/#HELMERT
10. Jaki T, Wolfsegger MJ. (2011). Estimation of pharmacokinetic parameters with the R package PK. *Pharm. Stat.*, 10:284–288. doi:10.1002/pst.449.
11. Schütz H, Labes D, Fuglsang A. (2014). Reference datasets for 2-treatment, 2-sequence, 2-period bioequivalence studies. *AAPS J.*, 16(6):1292–1297. doi:10.120 8/s12248-014-9661-0.
12. Labes D, Schuetz H, Lang B. (2018). PowerTOST: Power and Sample Size Based on Two One-Sided t-Tests (TOST) for (Bio)Equivalence Studies. R package version 1.4-7. https://CRAN.R-project.org/package=PowerTOST
13. Bae KS. (2018). BE: Bioequivalence Study Data Analysis. R package version 0.1.1. https://CRAN.R-project.org/package=BE
14. Sthda.com. (2019). *ggplot2 violin plot: Quick start guide—R software and data visualization—Easy Guides—Wiki—STHDA*. http://www.sthda.com/english/wiki/ggplot2-violin-plot-quick-start-guide-r-software-and-data-visualization [Accessed 26 July 2019].

15. Sthda.com. (2019). *One-Way ANOVA Test in R—Easy Guides—Wiki—STHDA.* http://www.sthda.com/english/wiki/one-way-anova-test-in-r [Accessed 27 July 2019].
16. Benjamini Y, Hochberg Y. (1995). Controlling the false discovery rate: A practical and powerful approach to multiple testing. *J. R. Stat. Soc. B*, 57(1):289–300.
17. Math.ucsd.edu. (2019). http://www.math.ucsd.edu/~rxu/math284/slect7.pdf [Accessed 28 July 2019].
18. Therneau T. (2015). *A Package for Survival Analysis in S.* version 2.38, https://CRAN.R-project.org/package=survival.
19. Lee Y, Molas M, Noh M. (2018). mdhglm: Multivariate Double Hierarchical Generalized Linear Models. R package version 1.8. https://CRAN.R-project.org/package=mdhglm
20. Bioconductor.org. (2019). http://www.bioconductor.org/packages//2.12/data/experiment/vignettes/estrogen/inst/doc/estrogen.pdf [Accessed 6 August 2019].
21. Csardi G, Nepusz T. (2006). The igraph software package for complex network research, InterJournal, Complex Systems 1695 http://igraph.org
22. "ggplot2: Quick Correlation Matrix Heatmap—R Software and Data Visualization." *STHDA*, www.sthda.com/english/wiki/ggplot2-quick-correlation-matrix-heatmap-r-software-and-data-visualization.
23. R-bloggers. (2019). *Forest Plot (with Horizontal Bands)*.https://www.r-bloggers.com/forest-plot-with-horizontal-bands/
24. Max Gordon and Thomas Lumley (2019). forestplot: Advanced Forest Plot Using 'grid' Graphics. R package version 1.9. https://CRAN.R-project.org/package=forestplot
25. Rizopoulos D, Verbeke G, Lesaffre E. (2009). Fully exponential laplace approximations for the joint modelling of survival and longitudinal data. *J. Royal Stat. Soc. B*, 71:637–654.
26. Rizopoulos D. (2010). JM: An R package for the joint modelling of longitudinal and time-to-event data. *J. Stat. Softw.*, 35(9):1–33. http://www.jstatsoft.org/v35/i09/
27. M3(R2) Nonclinical safety studies for the conduct of human clinical trials and marketing authorization for pharmaceuticals http://www.fda.gov/downloads/Drugs/GuidanceComplianceRegulatoryInformation/Guidances/UCM073246.pdf
28. WHO Technical Report Series 996, 2016, Annex 9. https://www.who.int/medicines/publications/pharmprep/WHO_TRS_996_annex09.pdf?ua=1

Section II

Predictive Biomarkers

7

Introduction

We start this chapter by differentiating between *prognostic biomarker* and *predictive biomarkers*. Prognostic biomarkers measure disease prognosis or are associated with the disease outcome without consideration to treatment. These markers are of primary interest for companies making diagnostic tests for detection of disease and/or disease severity and/or disease classification. They identify the likelihood of a clinical event. Predictive biomarkers measures are concerned with identifying patients who will respond (present favorable clinical outcome) to treatment. The same biomarker can be both prognostic and predictive, hence the terms are not mutually exclusive for a biomarker. In fact, a biomarker measured at baseline can be neither, either or both prognostic and predictive. Safety biomarkers are also predictive and measure the likelihood of a toxic event as a result of treatment. A prognostic biomarker may be of interest to a company making a pharmaceutical product, in order to screen patients who will qualify for entry into a clinical trial. In general, we will focus on predictive biomarkers and relevant statistical analyses in this part of the book.

7.1 Predictive Marker and Drug Co-development Paradigm

A companion diagnostic (CDx) test for a drug is a test for a predictive biomarker of the response of the drug in a patient. It is at the heart of personalized medicine. The Food and Drug Administration (FDA) is in the forefront of guiding the industry to co-develop the drug along with its companion diagnostic (CDx) where both products (not necessarily from the same company) follow a set regulatory pathway for approval.

According to the FDA,

> a companion diagnostic is a medical device, often an in vitro device, which provides information that is essential for the safe and effective use of a corresponding drug or biological product. The test helps a healthcare professional determine whether a particular therapeutic product's benefits to patients will outweigh any potential serious side effects or risks.

Companion diagnostics can:

- identify patients who are most likely to benefit from a particular therapeutic product
- identify patients likely to be at increased risk for serious side effects as a result of treatment with a particular therapeutic product
- monitor response to treatment with a particular therapeutic product for the purpose of adjusting treatment to achieve improved safety or effectiveness.

If the diagnostic test is inaccurate, then the treatment decision based on that test may not be optimal.

On July 31, 2014, the FDA issued 'Guidance for Industry: In Vitro Companion Diagnostic Devices', to help companies identify the need for companion diagnostics at an earlier stage in the drug development process and to plan for co-development of the drug and companion diagnostic test. The ultimate goal of the guidance is to stimulate early collaborations that will result in faster access to promising new treatments for patients living with serious and life-threatening diseases [32].

Let me illustrate the co-development paradigm by the graphic below [31]:

Drug Discovery	Preclinical Trials	Phase I Trials Clinical	Phase II Trials Clinical	Phase 3 Trials Clinical	Postmarket Surveillance
Parallel Co-Development of Drug and Diagnostic Test (Predictive Biomarker)					
Biomarker Development & Selection	Conduct Feasibility Studies	Build Prototype Assay	Analytical Validation	Clinical Validation	Clinical Utility

Even though the CDx studies and assay development do not have to be exactly in lock-step with the drug, the clinical validation of the CDx as a predictive biomarker for the drug being developed must be supported by the data obtained from the phase 3 clinical trial of the drug.

Let us now focus on the statistical analyses for assessing the drug response in the subgroup selected by the predictive biomarker.

7.2 Statistical Model for Predictive Biomarker with Continuous Clinical Endpoint

Statistically, let us represent the biomarker effects in terms of a linear model when the disease outcome is continuous:

$$E\left(Y \mid \text{Trt, BM}\right) = \beta_0 + \beta_{Trt} Trt + \beta_{BM} BM + \beta_{IX} Trt \times BM$$

- When $\beta_{BM} = 0$ and $\beta_{IX} = 0$: the marker is neither predictive or prognostic
- When $\beta_{BM} \neq 0$ and $\beta_{IX} = 0$: the marker is prognostic, but not
- When $\beta_{BM} = 0$ and $\beta_{IX} \neq 0$: the marker is predictive, but not prognostic
- When $\beta_{BM} \neq 0$ and $\beta_{IX} \neq 0$: the marker is both predictive and prognostic

Note, the interaction design given below in Figure 7.2 is necessary in order for the interaction effect above to be estimable. Also, note that for time to event outcome or binary response outcome, the linear model would be replaced by the appropriate regression model to estimate the interaction effect between the predictive biomarker and treatment. As mentioned before, in drug development context, where a biomarker is being considered with a companion diagnostic test (CDx) to determine the eligibility for entry into the trial for conditional entry or for stratification based on the marker value, we usually refer to it as a *predictive biomarker*. This is the context of this chapter in the book. Of course, it is possible to have prognostic biomarkers tested for other entry criteria and disease monitoring markers measured during the trial, but those are not part of our discussion here. Predictive biomarkers are measured in subjects at the baseline, that is, on entry to a clinical trial of a particular drug, sponsored by a pharmaceutical company.

As you can see from the general notation of the model above, it is essential to have at least a two-arm (treatment vs control) trial with biomarker assessments for subjects at entry to be available to determine its predictive utility of the treatment effect.

Numerous steps are taken in the journey of developing a drug through exploratory studies through phase III confirmatory studies; and co-developing a predictive biomarker for patient selection for ensuring the treatment effect of the drug is meaningful in selected patients, makes it atleast doubly complex. The benefits are tremendous however, when the treatment works in the selected group of patients only. As mentioned before, the process above is dubbed as the *drug–diagnostic co-development model*, which involves the parallel development of the drug and the diagnostic test for the predictive biomarker. This is a multidisciplinary task where statisticians play a key role in the pharma industry. In fact, in a large company, several statisticians may be involved in the life cycle of a drug–diagnostic co-development model as it spans multiple years.

Recent advances in statistical and scientific methods have created support for shortening the process so that drugs that are suitable for a subgroup, and not for all subjects afflicted with the disease, appear in the market sooner rather than later. To this end, pharmaceutical industry, academia, and regulatory authorities have to rapidly develop methods and guidance to facilitate this era of precision or personalized medicine.

7.3 Three Basic Designs for Predictive Biomarker Enabled Trial

There are many proposed designs for drug development with a predictive biomarker, but we will focus mainly on the analysis of data on such trials rather than the design here. Before we delve in the analysis issues, it is worth noting that the designs proposed are roughly in three categories:

- biomarker identified subgroup
- biomarker stratified design
- biomarker adaptive design

Figure 7.1 is a schematic for the *biomarker identified subgroup* design. Figure 7.2 is a schematic for *biomarker stratified design*. Figure 7.3 is a schematic for *biomarker adaptive design*.

There are many variations of these basic three types. Antoniou [8] et al. have presented a great summary of strategies for nonadaptive Phase II and Phase III clinical trial designs with biomarkers. Moreover, their review article presents sample size formulae for all the designs. Another well-written review of biomarker integrated trial designs is the paper by Buyse et al. [21].

For the first type of design, biomarker identified subgroup, I refer to designing a trial for only the biomarker-positive patients (BM+). This means that the biomarker cutoff is known, which means it is known with scientific evidence that the treatment agent has minimal

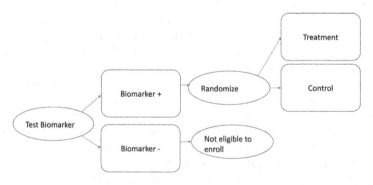

FIGURE 7.1
Biomarker identified design (targeted design).

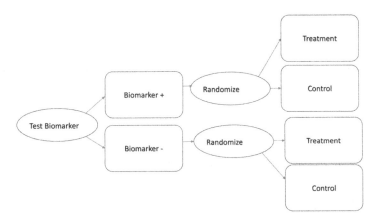

FIGURE 7.2
Biomarker stratified design (interaction design).

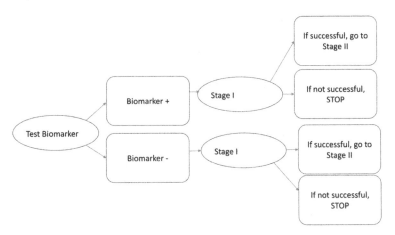

FIGURE 7.3
Biomarker adaptive design.

or no effect (or even deleterious effect) in the biomarker-negative (BM−) subgroup. Therefore, the Phase II or III trial will proceed in the BM+ subgroup only. Alternatively, one may refine the cut point of the biomarker through a BM+ subgroup, where a few candidate cut points may be tested in this design, but the biomarker-negative subgroup is largely excluded. Two of the classic examples for biomarker identified subgroup only clinical trials are (i) Herceptin in HER2+ breast cancer patients [9] and (ii) Vemurafenib for BRAF V600E mutation in melanoma patients [10]. We will not discuss this design further.

For the second type of design, the biomarker stratified design, I address a number of statistical issues for proof-of-concept and confirmatory trials in Chapters 8 and 9, respectively of this part of the book.

For the third type of design, the biomarker adaptive design, I discuss statistical methodology that is evolving rapidly to address issues, like learning the biomarker cut points (for determining subgroups) for one or multiple biomarkers, while confirming treatment effects defined by those subgroups in the same trial or in seamless combination trials.

With the general sketch of the three types of designs out of the way, I will now focus on statistical issues arising in these designs, where patients of biomarker-positive and -negative groups are present. However, we do need patients' biomarker value to be available at the time of randomization via a validated test. By validated test, I mean a test with completed analytical validation with acceptable accuracy, sensitivity, and specificity.

In the stratified design, the biomarker cut point is known and subjects in both BM+ and BM− subgroups are randomized to either treatment or control regimen. The reason BM− subgroup is included because they may derive treatment benefit as well or the treatment effect in the overall population may be acceptable. The main statistical issue here is testing endpoint(s) multiple times.

Furthermore, I discuss the case where the biomarker is continuous and a threshold (or cutoff or cut point) for dichotomization is not known. Assuming the biomarker has a monotonically increasing relationship with treatment outcome, I discuss issues of cut point determination in Chapters 4 and 5 in this part of the book, for a continuous biomarker with respect to treatment–biomarker interaction, as well as biomarker group vs its complement group. In trials where we need to determine the biomarker threshold, we recruit all comers, randomize them to treatment and control regimens, and study the appropriate cutoff for the biomarker among all subjects in the clinical trial. It might take time to refine and establish the cutoff over multiple clinical trials. For example, the cutoff can be narrowed down to two choices in a proof-of-concept trial and ultimately proved in a confirmatory trial. Or, the threshold identification and treatment effect confirmation can be done in a seamless Phase II/III trial.

Learning and refining the cut point for a continuous biomarker can proceed up until Phase III, or even Phase IV studies, if necessary.

8

Operational Characteristics of Proof-of-Concept Trials with Biomarker-Positive and -Negative Subgroups

Often, in Proof-of-Concept (PoC) studies (typically Phase 2), a statistician is asked to fill out the operational characteristics of several design options for biomarker subgroups and the overall population. Here, I am referring to a dichotomous biomarker (threshold or cutoff known), and the objective of the PoC study would be to establish that the therapeutic agent is active in the biomarker-positive (BM+) group and less active in the overall population.

In addition to the cutoff for the biomarker positivity (negativity), I assume that the prevalence of the marker-positive population is known at the time of designing the clinical trial. While it is generally assumed that treatment effect in BM+ group is higher, clear evidence does not exist that the agent is not active in the biomarker-negative subgroup. Hence, the justification for doing a confirmatory trial in the marker-positive subgroup needs to be established. Alternatively, the PoC study will guide us to do the confirmatory trial in all subjects.

I made the following assumptions about the BM+ group and the overall population in preparation for (i) the recruitment and study duration and (ii) power calculations in the R package 'rpact' [2] (Table 8.1).

8.1 Recruitment and Study Duration of Marker Subgroup and Overall Population

The strategy for planning a trial where we see a treatment effect in the BM+ group, as well as in the overall population, is about synchronizing the two designs so that study duration and recruitment end at about the same time. You can use any commercially available sample size calculation software to design it using this same strategy shown below. However, we will use the validated R package, 'rpact', which is available for free.

TABLE 8.1

Assumptions about the BM+ Group and the Overall Population

	Biomarker Positive	Biomarker Negative	Overall
Prevalence	1/3	2/3	
Hazard ratio	0.5	1	0.8
Lambda2=hazard rate in placebo group	Log(2)/12	Log(2)/20	Log(2)/17.33
Lambda1=hazard rate in treated group	Log(2)/24	Log(2)/20	Log(2)/20.33
Alpha One-sided	0.05		0.1
Power	0.8		0.65

The R code is given below and follows the examples shown in the handy vignettes accompanying the package:

```
# set up data frame which contains sample sizes and
corresponding durations
sampleSizeDuration <- data.frame(          #BM positive
  maxNumberSubjects=c(75,100,125,150,175),
  accrualTime=NA,
  studyDuration=NA)
# calculate recruitment and study duration for each sample size
for (i in 1:nrow(sampleSizeDuration)){
  sampleSizeResult <- getSampleSizeSurvival(
    sided = 1,alpha = 0.05,beta = 0.2,
    lambda2 = log(2)/12,hazardRatio = .5,
    dropoutRate1 = 0.08, dropoutRate2 = 0.025,dropoutTime = 18,
    accrualTime = c(0,1,2,3,4,5,6),
    accrualIntensity = c(2,4,6,8,10,12,14),
    maxNumberOfSubjects =
sampleSizeDuration$maxNumberSubjects[i])
  sampleSizeDuration$accrualTime[i] <-
sampleSizeResult$totalAccrualTime
  sampleSizeDuration$studyDuration[i] <-
sampleSizeResult$maxStudyDuration
}

sampleSizeDuration2 <- data.frame( #Overall
  maxNumberSubjects=c(225,300,375,450,525),
  accrualTime=NA,
  studyDuration=NA)
# calculate recruitment and study duration for each sample size
for (i in 1:nrow(sampleSizeDuration2)){
  sampleSizeResult2 <- getSampleSizeSurvival(
    sided = 1,alpha = 0.1,beta = 0.35,
    lambda2 = log(2)/16,hazardRatio = exp(log(.5)*1/3 +
log(1)*2/3),
```

```
    dropoutRate1 = 0.05, dropoutRate2 = 0.025,dropoutTime = 18,
    accrualTime = c(0,1,2,3,4,5,6),
    accrualIntensity = c(6,12,18,24,30,36,42),
    maxNumberOfSubjects =
sampleSizeDuration2$maxNumberSubjects[i])
  sampleSizeDuration2$accrualTime[i] <-
sampleSizeResult2$totalAccrualTime
  sampleSizeDuration2$studyDuration[i] <-
sampleSizeResult2$maxStudyDuration
}
```

8.1.1 Operational Characteristics of the BM+ Group

The operational characteristics of the **marker-positive subgroup** are given in 'sampleSizeResult' and displayed as follows:

Design plan parameters and output for survival data:

Design parameters:
    Significance level: 0.0500
    Type II error rate: 0.2
    Test: one-sided

User defined parameters:
    Lambda (2): 0.0578
    Hazard ratio: 0.500
    Maximum number of subjects: 175.0
    Event time: 12
    Accrual intensity: 2.0, 4.0, 6.0, 8.0, 10.0, 12.0, 14.0
    Drop-out rate (1): 0.080
    Drop-out rate (2): 0.025
    Drop-out time: 18.00

Default parameters:
    Type of computation: Schoenfeld
    Theta H0: 1
    Planned allocation ratio: 1
    Piecewise survival times: 0.00

Sample size and output:
    Direction upper: FALSE
    pi (1): 0.293

pi (2): 0.500
Median (1): 24.0
Median (2): 12.0
Lambda (1): 0.0289
Number of events: 51.5
Accrual time: 1.00, 2.00, 3.00, 4.00, 5.00, 6.00, 15.50
Total accrual time: 15.50
Follow up time: 2.26
Calculate follow up time: TRUE
Number of subjects fixed: 175.0
Number of subjects fixed (1): 87.5
Number of subjects fixed (2): 87.5
Analysis times: 17.76
Study duration: 17.76
Critical values (effect scale): 0.632
Local one-sided significance levels: 0.0500

We see that d = 50 events are necessary in the subgroup for 80% power in detecting a hazard ratio of 0.5. The study duration is calculated to be about 1.5 years and accrual continues until about 1.25 years.

8.1.2 Operational Characteristics of the Overall Population

The operational characteristics of the **overall population** are given in 'sampleSizeResult2' and displayed as follows:

```
> sampleSizeResult2
```

Design plan parameters and output for survival data:

Design parameters:
    Significance level: 0.1000
    Type II error rate: 0.35
    Test: one-sided

User defined parameters:
    Lambda (2): 0.040
    Hazard ratio: 0.794
    Maximum number of subjects: 525.0

Event time: 12

Accrual intensity: 6.0, 12.0, 18.0, 24.0, 30.0, 36.0, 42.0

Drop-out rate (1): 0.050

Drop-out rate (2): 0.025

Drop-out time: 18.00

Default parameters:

Type of computation: Schoenfeld

Theta H0: 1

Planned allocation ratio: 1

Piecewise survival times: 0.00

Sample size and output:

Direction upper: FALSE

pi (1): 0.317

pi (2): 0.381

Median (1): 21.8

Median (2): 17.3

Lambda (1): 0.0317

Number of events: 208.2

Accrual time: 1.00, 2.00, 3.00, 4.00, 5.00, 6.00, 15.50

Total accrual time: 15.50

Follow up time: 8.25

Calculate follow up time: TRUE

Number of subjects fixed: 525.0

Number of subjects fixed (1): 262.5

Number of subjects fixed (2): 262.5

Analysis times: 23.75

Study duration: 23.75

Critical values (effect scale): 0.837

Local one-sided significance levels: 0.1000

We see that d = 210 events are necessary overall for 65% power in detecting a hazard ratio of 0.8. The study duration is calculated to be 1.75 years and accrual continues until 1.25 years.

These two tables are approximately synchronized, with the overall population driving the study duration prediction to be 24 months and maximum number of subjects to be 525 (i.e., number in BM+ group = 175).

8.1.3 Plots of the BM+ Group and Overall Population

The R code below will make a nice visual plot of the results above:

```
#BM pos
plot(sampleSizeDuration$maxNumberSubjects,
    sampleSizeDuration$studyDuration,type="l",
    xlab="Total sample size",
    ylab="Duration (months)",

    main="Recruitment and study duration vs sample size",

ylim=c(0,max(sampleSizeDuration2$studyDuration)),xlim=c
(50,600),
    col="grey",lwd=1.5)
lines(sampleSizeDuration$maxNumberSubjects,
    sampleSizeDuration$accrualTime,col="black",lwd=1.5)
legend(x=350,y=100,cex=.5,
    legend=c("BM+ : Study duration under H1",
            "BM+ : Recruitment duration"),
    col=c("grey","black"),lty=1,lwd=1.5)

#Overall
lines(sampleSizeDuration2$maxNumberSubjects,
    sampleSizeDuration2$studyDuration,lty=2,
    col="gray",lwd=1.5)
lines(sampleSizeDuration2$maxNumberSubjects,
    sampleSizeDuration2$accrualTime,col="black",lwd=1.5,
lty=2)
legend(x=350,y=80,cex=.5,
    legend=c("Overall: Study duration under H1",
            "Overall: Recruitment duration"),
    col=c("grey","black"),lty=2,lwd=1.5)
abline(h=24)
```

The curves on the left in Figure 8.1 are for the BM+ group and those on the right are for the overall population.

We see in Figure 8.1 that the accrual time is 15.5 months in both the marker-positive subgroup and overall population; it is possible to achieve the study duration of 24 months when the sample size in the overall population is 525.

You can vary the power, alpha, and other input parameters to suit the design needs of your PoC trial.

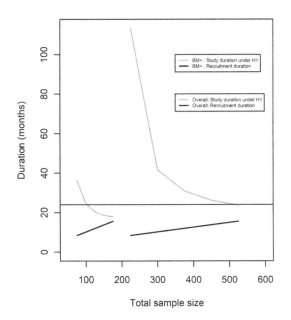

FIGURE 8.1
Recruitment and study duration vs sample size.

8.2 Power Curves for Marker Subgroup and Overall Population

The power curves for both populations are plotted in Figure 8.2 for different hazard ratios on the x-axis. The BM+ subgroup power curves are on the *right*; the overall population curves are on the *left*; for each population, the different curves account for varying number of events.

The horizontal lines are drawn at 80% power for the marker subgroup and 65% power for the overall population. The bottom-most power curve from the bottom for the marker-positive subgroup on the right achieves 80% power for detecting a hazard ratio of 0.5 (or $1/0.5 = 2$) with d = 65. The number of events was calculated as $\dfrac{\left(\dfrac{z_\alpha + z_\beta}{2}\right)^2}{\pi_1 \pi_2 (\log HR)^2}$ for input into the function getPowerSurvival():

```
pow=getPowerSurvival(design = des, hazardRatio=haz,
      maxNumberOfEvents = nevts[i], maxNumberOfSubjects = n[i],
      lambda2=log(2)/medn, directionUpper = TRUE)
```

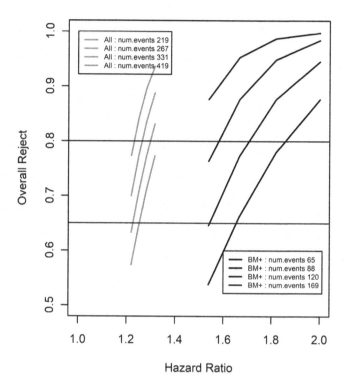

FIGURE 8.2
Power vs hazard ratio.

We achieve 65% power for detecting a hazard ratio of 0.8 with d = 219 in the overall population. As you can see, these numbers are in agreement with the previous plots that gave us feasible recruitment and accrual schedules.

The R package 'rpact' also contains functions for calculating operational characteristics for group sequential designs with continuous and binary response. The strategy shown above can also be applied in those cases. Note that an interim analysis is not needed to use this package; however, it is flexible enough to accommodate a multistage, biomarker subgroup, and overall population design, in order to facilitate several formal comparisons. It is useful to read the vignettes that are generously provided by the consortium that produced this validated R package.

8.3 Multiple Testing for BM+ Subgroup and Overall Population

Since we are looking at two endpoints in this PoC trial setting, we want to implement a strategy for testing both hypotheses for statistical significance. PoC trials are usually smaller in size than confirmatory trials, thus I have used an overall level of alpha of 0.1 for this example I posed above. There are several ways to account for testing two endpoints, but here I employ the strategy of looking at the two univariate P values.

Much has been written about combining m independent P values in the statistical literature for clinical trials. The simplest of course in the Bonferroni correction. If we are testing m equally weighted hypotheses $H_1, H_2, ..., H_m$, then the procedure will reject H_k if $p_k \leq \frac{\alpha}{m}$. This is quite conservative and quite unlikely to be met in the overall population in our example, since the majority of the subjects are in the biomarker-negative subgroup. This attenuates the hazard ratio for the overall population to 0.8.

Instead, our strategy has been to use the Holm procedure [3], which involves stepwise testing. Since we are equally weighting the BM+ group and the overall population hypothesis, we simply

- Test the most significant P value (BM+ subgroup) against $\frac{\alpha}{m}$ or $\frac{0.1}{2} = 0.05$; if it rejects, we go to the step below
- Test the less significant P value (overall population) against $\frac{\alpha}{(m-k+1)} = \frac{0.1}{2-2+1} = 0.1$; if it rejects, we can see evidence of statistical significance of the treatment effect at alpha = 0.1 level for the overall population.

9

A Framework for Testing Biomarker Subgroups in Confirmatory Trials

As mentioned before, a dichotomous *predictive* biomarker separating positive and negative subgroups of patients is assumed to be available through a companion diagnostic test (CDx) with well-established sensitivity, specificity and overall accuracy before undertaking the confirmatory trial.

For the purposes of this chapter, we assume that a confirmatory trial is designed for making joint inference on the biomarker-positive (BM+) subpopulation (those presumed to have high response to treatment) and the overall population. If it is known that there is no treatment effect in the biomarker negative subgroup, then a confirmatory trial should be carried out in the BM+ subgroup of patients only.

For the rest of this chapter, we assume that at the time of designing the confirmatory trial for the drug, it is *not* known with statistical confidence that only the BM+ subgroup will respond to treatment.

This means that we have uncertainty around the treatment effect in the biomarker-negative subgroup; however, we have evidence that the drug may be active in the BM+ and possibly in the overall population. When we have the opportunity to confirm a treatment effect separately by running two independent trials in the positive and negative subpopulations, the problems of multiplicity adjustments disappear [4]. On the other hand, if we ignore the biomarker effect and run one trial on subjects from the overall population to confirm the treatment effect, then the sponsor is taking a huge risk. Ultimately, the sponsor is responsible for adequately powering the trial for the population(s) of interest. There are several instances in the pharmaceutical industry, where ignoring the biomarker effect has led to a failure to reject the null hypothesis of no treatment effect in the overall population. The reason is that subjects from the whole population are too heterogeneous in their drug response.

9.1 Co-primary Testing: The Overall Population and BM+ Group for Efficacy

At times, both the treatment effects in the BM+ subgroup and overall population are of interest to test as co-primary endpoints. The objective is to show a treatment effect in both. Alternatively, one of the hypothesis can be tested as

primary and the other as secondary, but then the study is not formally pow-
ered for testing both. Having both tests listed as co-primary accounts for that.

Testing the co-primary endpoints is an *intersection–union* test [6]. This test
does not inflate the type I error rate. This means each of the endpoints can be
tested at the same significance level of α. However, the hypotheses inflate the
type II error rate and reduce the power of the test. By properly accounting for
the type II error, you will inflate the sample size of the trial. Power will also
depend on the magnitude of the treatment effects in each of the co-primary
endpoints. The R package *'mpe'* implements this design for generating the
necessary sample sizes.

9.2 Multiple Primary Testing: The Overall
Population and BM+ Group for Efficacy

In cases of testing BM+, BM−, and overall populations, it is more often that
we will test the hypothesis as a *union–intersection* test [6]. This means that
we will consider a win if any of the hypothesis is rejected (or at least one
is rejected). We have a closed testing procedure for H_{BM-}, H_{BM+}, and $H_{\forall}$.
This procedure rejects the intersection hypothesis at an adjusted alpha level
and, if rejected, tests the other hypotheses at level α. This amounts to testing
the most significant P value or the maximal t statistics against the adjusted
α level or critical value.

There are several strategies to consider here, and I will mention only a few:

1. Fixed Sequence Testing

   This is more powerful than other procedures when the ordering of
   each intersecting hypothesis is fixed and known.

2. Bonferroni procedure for multiple testing can be applied to the
   closed testing setting where each of the marginal P values can be
   tested against the α level of $\frac{\alpha}{k}$, where k = # of elemental hypotheses.

3. The Hochberg and Holm procedure can be used as well. For detailed
   examples, refer to lecture notes (see Mehta [7], Dmitrienko [6], or
   Halabi [5]).

4. The Dunnett procedure, which is described below.

Before we describe the Dunnett procedure, which lets us account for the correlation between the BM+ and overall population, it is helpful to state the
premise for coming up with a strategy for testing the biomarker subgroups.
Glimm and Di Scala [3] summarizes a few strategies for the scenarios in
which a confirmatory trial is necessary to make an inference on the BM+
and the overall population. Again, I assume that the cutoff or threshold for

the biomarker dichotomization is known and established. Or, perhaps the biomarker is dichotomous in nature, like when a genetic mutation is present or absent. (Later chapters address the issues of finding the cutoff for a continuous marker separately.)

The strategy of testing a treatment effect in the overall population and the BM+ subgroup is the main focus of this chapter. It is assumed that the magnitude of the treatment effect in the BM+ group is larger than that of the whole population. Glimm et al. recommend the hierarchical strategy of testing as following:

- Test overall population ($\forall$) and then BM+ or
- Test BM+ and then overall population ($\forall$)

They recommend when there is high value in maintaining all-comers, the first strategy is followed; when there is high confidence in the BM+ subgroup, the second strategy is appropriate.

9.2.1 Dunnett Procedure

We assume that you can estimate the correlation between the test statistics, which makes the Dunnett procedure more powerful than a Bonferroni correction. The statistical framework is set up by Glimm et al. [3] and mentioned above. The underlying basis is that the test statistics are normally distributed. In oncology, for example, where the log rank test statistic or the regression coefficient from the Cox proportional hazards model are normally distributed. Therefore, this assumption is useful in many settings. The framework they introduce is based on contrast estimation and statistical hypothesis testing in ANOVA models. The general null hypothesis is $H_0 = H_{BM+} \cap H_{BM-} \cap H_\forall$ which is a level α test where $1 - P_{H_0}(t_s \leq Q_s$ for all $s) = \alpha$. The cumulative distribution function of $P(t_s \leq Q_s$ for all $s)$ under the null and any alternative hypothesis is a multivariate normal or central t distribution. This makes the procedure more powerful than Bonferroni. In this procedure, we have to derive critical values and P values from this multivariate distribution to test our hypotheses of interest. Glimm et al. explain that setting the critical values $Q_{BM+} = Q_\forall$ results in the ordinary Dunnett's procedure; and setting differential weights leads us to a weighted Dunnett's test procedure. The weighted Dunnett procedure and the corresponding R code are presented by Glimm [5].

9.2.2 Dunnett Procedure—Example

Halabi et al. [5] give a nice example of the BELLE-4 Study in metastatic breast cancer in their book, which we will use here for illustrative purposes.

Let the test statistics for the BM+ and the overall population be denoted as $(t_{BM+}, t_\forall)$. Then, the joint distribution of $(t_{BM+}, t_\forall)^T$ is approximately bivariate normal with mean $(0,0)^T$ and variance–covariance matrix $\begin{pmatrix} 1 & \rho \\ \rho & 1 \end{pmatrix}$. The correlation can be approximated with the ratio of the number of events in the two populations, $\frac{d_{BM+}}{d_V}$. Note the number of events in the two groups is a good approximation since the subgroup is part of the overall population; moreover, this covariance matrix holds when the treatment effects are standardized and the general null hypothesis that treatment has no effect.

The BELLE-4 Study had 131 progression events overall and 42 in the PI3K-activated subgroup.

First, we set up the correlation matrix in R. Second, we get the critical value for the test:

```
> corr=(1-sqrt(42/131))*diag(2)+sqrt(42/131)
> Q= qmvnorm(.95,tail="both",corr=corr)$quantile
```

Q is the one-sided critical value for the Dunnett's test we perform. The critical value returned is 2.203844, which is less than the Bonferroni corrected critical score of 2.24.

The procedure states that the maximum of the (t_{BM+}, t_V) must be equal to greater than Q for the test to reject the global hypotheses.

Third, we can compute the adjusted P value (one-sided and two-sided) by direct numerical integration of the bivariate normal density in R as follows:

```
>1-pmvnorm(upper=c(t_F,t_F), lower=c(-Inf,-Inf),corr=corr,)
>1-pmvnorm(upper=c(t_A,t_A), lower=c(-t_A,-t_A),corr=corr)[[1]]
```

The R function 'pmvnorm' is used; you can use R function 'pmvt' for multivariate t distribution if you need. The R code is available from Glimm et al. [3].

9.2.2.1 Power Calculations

For power calculations in a confirmatory trial, you may use specialized, commercial power calculation software to do sample size calculations. However, you can also use R or you can use R to double-check your sample size calculations. Given the framework set up by Glimm et al. [3], the power curves are simple to generate.

Let us consider the number of events in the overall population to vary between 100 and 200, also the HR in the overall population to be 0.8 and the HR in the BM+ subgroup to be 0.65. The standard error for each log(HR) can be estimated under the null as $\sqrt{\frac{1}{d_{s,Trt}} + \frac{1}{d_{s,Ctrl}}} = \sqrt{\frac{2}{d_s}}$.

The R code for generating the power curves is given below.

```
d.all=seq(100,200,5)
d.BM.pos=round(d.all*.33)
```

```
pow=NULL
for (i in 1:length(d.all)){
  pow=c(pow,1-pmvnorm(lower=-Q,upper=Q,
mean=c(log(.8)/sqrt(2/d.all[i]),log(.65)/sqrt(2/d. BM.
pos[i])), corr=corr)[[1]])
}
plot(pow,d.all,xlim=c(.4,1),type="o",
      main="Power via parametric Dunnett
procedure",xlab="power",ylab="# events overall")
par(new=TRUE)
plot(pow,d.BM.pos,col=2, type = "l", xaxt = "n",yaxt="n",
      ylab = "", xlab = "")
axis(side = 4)
mtext("#events BM+", side = 4)
```

The power of parametric Dunnett procedure is shown below, and we see that 80% power in the overall population is not reached given the sample sizes, marker prevalence, and standardized effect I chose.

Figure 9.1 shows the power curve of the overall population in the left, and the BM+ subgroup on the right.

Note that many statisticians will choose to code the full operational characteristics in R for the trial, but this gives useful calculations for sample size when designing the study. So this code could be a starting point for your needs.

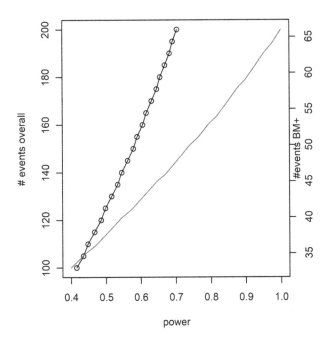

FIGURE 9.1
Power via parametric Dunnett procedure.

10

Cutoff Determination of Continuous Predictive Biomarker for a Biomarker–Treatment Interaction

When the cutoff (threshold) for dichotomizing a continuous biomarker is not known, we must use statistical methods to investigate the correct threshold concurrently with testing for treatment effect in the subgroups, as well as the overall population, and adjust for multiple comparisons.

There are two approaches to finding cut points for continuous, predictive biomarkers:

- The first approach is where many have worked on testing treatment effect in multiple marker-defined subgroups.
- Second approach is where statisticians have focused on looking at marker positive subgroup(s) vs the complement of the group with the objective to optimize the Phase III design as to whether or not to include all comers [1].

We discuss the *first approach* in this chapter and the *second approach* in the following chapter (Chapter 11).

Haller et al. [11] have done a comprehensive review of various methods in the literature for cut point determination for continuous predictive biomarkers with respect to biomarker–treatment interaction. The authors compare a few of the popular methods including the (i) median split, (ii) the quartile split, and (iii) the optimal split and (iv) Subpopulation Treatment Effect Pattern Plot (STEPP) method, and others for few different scenarios. In most of the prevalent scenarios that we encounter in modeling biomarker influence on treatment, these methods do well. For example, they simulated data, including biomarker, time-to-event outcome, and treatment variables, for the following scenarios:

- the biomarker is not associated with the risk of event irrespective of treatment
- the biomarker is prognostic and has a comparable effect on both treatment groups, with no interaction effect

- the biomarker has a linear interaction with treatment effect on risk of event
- the biomarker has a truly qualitative treatment (monotonic, but not linear) interaction, which means that in the negative group, there is minimal or no effect; however, there is an effect in the positive subgroup

The methods mentioned above did well in the above prevalent scenarios in detecting the threshold. Even though dichotomizing a marker generally leads to loss of statistical power, still it is necessary to identify the right group of subjects at times. If a marker has a truly linear interaction effect with treatment, then dichotomizing does not have any utility.

More advanced methods are required for more complex scenarios, like nonlinear interactions, or other shapes of biomarker treatment effect function over biomarker values in the two treatment groups. We will proceed below with the assumption that the biomarker–treatment interaction is one of the four prevalent scenarios above.

10.1 Splitting a Continuous Predictive Biomarker

The first method of *median split* is simply dividing the overall population into two halves at the median value of the biomarker. The *quartile split* produces a categorical biomarker. The *optimal split* considers all possible values (minus the extremes, like the upper and lower 10%) and chooses the cut point where the test statistics for the interaction term (treatment × biomarker group) is maximized (see section 7.2 for the linear regression model). We will discuss this method further here. Hothorn and Lausen [12] introduced the exact distribution methodology for maximally selected rank statistics, which gives as the ability to adjust the P value and effect sizes for making multiple comparisons. In addition to this method, there are two computational procedures for correcting P values and adjusting treatment effect sizes that I want to discuss: nonparametric bootstrap and Bayesian biomarker threshold models. Even though there are several other algorithms, we will focus on these two procedures in our example below.

Before we proceed to give details about these two computational procedures for the *optimal split* method with time-to-event data, I want to mention that the STEPP method introduced by Bonetti and Gelber [13] is also used quite a bit in several publications. This method explores the treatment–covariate interactions in survival or generalized linear model (GLM) for continuous, binomial, and count data arising from two or more treatment arms of a clinical trial. A permutation distribution approach to inference is implemented, based on permuting the covariate values within each treatment group. This procedure is implemented via the R package 'stepp' [14] and is readily available for finding biomarker cut points for continuous, binary, and time-to-event outcomes. I have not included this in the example below, but the reader can easily explore this method on her own from the package manual.

10.2 The Optimal Split Method of Dichotomizing Continuous Biomarker for Predicting Treatment Effect

The *optimal split* method is popular for finding the threshold of a continuous biomarker in the predictive setting. There are quite a few procedures and R packages for automating cut point selection in the prognostic setting, which are very helpful in developing diagnostic biomarkers. We are interested, however, in finding which cut point determines the optimal or maximized *treatment* effect for the biomarker identified subgroup in the drug development setting.

As mentioned before, if you are considering very few (2–4) cut points, you can use Bonferroni, Holm, or other methods to correct the P value for testing the treat by biomarker group interaction effect. For considering multiple cut points in the range of biomarker expression values, the asymptotic distribution proposed by Lausen [7] is available via their R package 'maxstat' [15] to adjust the P values and treatment effects. Note, multiple testing not only inflates the P value but also biases the treatment effect upward. It would be incorrect to report the unadjusted P value or treatment effect estimate since the estimates do not account for multiple looks. The problem, however, is that the package implements the correction in the prognostic setting, not in the predictive setting, for one or more biomarkers.

To this end, first, we illustrate the use of nonparametric bootstrap procedure to obtain the corrected treatment effect and confidence interval in the predictive setting for the *'optimal split'* procedure. Second, we mention a second, Bayesian method for optimal cut point selection. Even though this example is about survival analysis with time-to-event outcome, the methods and code will work for statistical models of treatment–biomarker interaction with continuous, binary, and categorical disease outcomes.

10.2.1 Survival Endpoint Model

Let T_i and C_i be the potential failure and censoring times for patient i in the study, respectively. Let $\delta_i = I(T_i < C_i)$ be a survival status indicator and $U_i = \min(T_i, C_i)$ the observed failure or censoring time, whichever occurs first.

Let $z_i = 1$ be the treatment indicator taking value 0 or 1 if patient i is assigned to a control or a new treatment group.

In addition, x_i is a continuous, predictive biomarker variable.

Given a threshold parameter ii for the biomarker variable x_i, the following proportional hazards model for the hazard function $\lambda(t)$ of the survival time T_i can be used to assess the treatment effect on the subset defined by the threshold,

$$\lambda(t \mid z_i, x_i, ii; \beta) = \lambda_0(t) \exp\{\beta_1 z_i + \beta_2 I(x_i > ii) + \beta_3 z_i I(x_i > ii)\}$$

where $\lambda_0(t)$ is the baseline hazard function.

With column vectors $Z_i(ii) = [z_i, I(x_i > ii), z_i I(x_i > ii)]'$ and $\beta = [\beta_1, \beta_2, \beta_3]'$, we can express the above model as $\lambda_0(t) \exp\{Z_i'(ii)\beta\}$.

We need to estimate the unknown parameter ii from a set of candidate cut points, ix. We assume a monotonic relationship between the biomarker values and treatment effect. In particular, we will assume that the shape of the biomarker–treatment effect curve is S shaped, or that the treatment effect is close to NULL in the biomarker-negative subgroup and achieves a positive magnitude in the biomarker-positive subgroup. The procedure described below will work for different shapes of biomarker–treatment effect curve.

The R functions I use below for obtaining the nonparametric bootstrap confidence intervals are derived in Morrison and Simon [16]. The authors present a parametric and a nonparametric bootstrap algorithm, with the latter being appropriate for our setting of subgroup selection. Algorithm #3 presented by the authors addresses the 'optimal splitting' problem directly, since the test statistics at different biomarker thresholds are correlated. Morrison et al. show that parametric bootstrap methods are not appropriate for data with complex dependence structures and/or for estimators without a known asymptotic distribution.

10.2.2 R Code for Cut Point Selection: Bootstrap Method

First, we download the biomarker threshold survival model with a single cut point generated in R package 'bhm' [12–14]. I will discuss this package at the end of this section. Second, I follow the set up suggested by Harrison [15] for estimating treatment effects in nested subgroups. I consider 50 values within the 20th and 80th percentiles of the biomarker. The vignette provided by Harrison makes it very easy to set up the model and get the interaction effect on hazard ratio and confidence intervals from the nonparametric bootstrap method for a sequence of candidate cut points:

```
library(bhm) #load Bayesian biomarker threshold
model (Chen et al) for comparison
library(rcc) #Threshold and bootstrapping by Jean Morrison
library(rccSims)
```

```
#First create the data per R package 'bhm'
n = 300
b = c(0.5, 1, 1.5)
data = surv.gendat(n, c0 = 0.40, beta = b)
age = runif(n, 0, 1)*100
tm = data[, 1]
status = data[, 2]
trt = data[, 3]
ki67 = data[, 4]
## fit a biomarker threshold survival model with one single
cut point
fit = bhm(Surv(tm, status)~ki67+trt+age, interaction = TRUE,
B=5, R=10)
print(fit) #This is the benchmark for the algorithm below
plot(fit)

#Now start processing the data for use with R package 'rcc'
n.cutpoints=50
quantile(data[,4],probs=seq(.2,.8,length.out=n.cutpoints))
->cutpoints
ix <- sapply(cutpoints, FUN=function(th){as.numeric(data[,4]
>= th)})

stats <- apply(ix, MARGIN=2, FUN=function(ii){
  f <- coxph(Surv(data[,1],data[,2])~data[,3]*ii)
  summary(f)$coeff[3,c(1,3,4)]
})

stats <- data.frame(matrix(unlist(stats), byrow=TRUE, ncol=3))

names(stats) <- c("beta", "se", "tstat")
stats$cutpoint <- cutpoints
j <- order(abs(stats$tstat), decreasing=TRUE)
stats$rank <- match(1:nrow(stats), j)
head(stats)

mydata <- cbind(data, ix)
analysis.func <- function(data){
#   y <- data[,4]
#   trt <- data[,1]
  stats <- apply(data[, 5:(n.cutpoints + 4)], MARGIN=2,
FUN=function(ii){
    f <- coxph(Surv(data[,1],data[,2])~data[,3]*ii)
    if(nrow(summary(f)$coefficients) < 3) return(rep(0, 3))
    summary(f)$coeff[3,c(1,3,4)]
  })
  stats <- data.frame(matrix(unlist(stats), byrow=TRUE,
  ncol=3))
  names(stats) <- c("estimate", "se", "statistic")
```

```
   return(stats)
}
ci.nonpar <- nonpar_bs_ci(data=mydata, analysis.func=analysis.
func, n.rep=500, parallel=TRUE)
#Find the cutpoint where max diff (drop) in test-statistics
occurs
plotCI(cutpoints,ci.nonpar$debiased.est,ui=ci.nonpar$ci.upper,
li=ci.nonpar$ci.lower)
idx=which.max(abs(diff(ci.nonpar[,6],lag=1)))
abline(v=cutpoints[idx],col="darkgrey",lwd=2,lty=2)

#End
```

The optimal threshold is identified as

```
> cutpoints[idx]
54.28571%
0.3533764
```

Plotting the adjusted hazard ratio estimates and confidence interval shows the threshold where there is the biggest change in hazard ratio between the biomarker-positive and -negative subgroups (Figure 10.1).

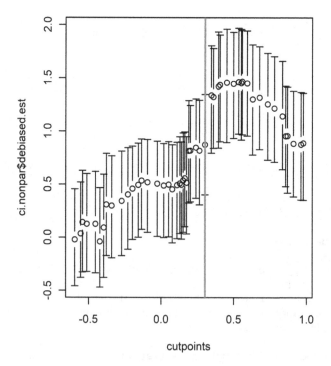

FIGURE 10.1
Adjusted hazard ratio and confidence interval for different cutpoints of the biomarker.

10.2.3 Cut Point Selection: R Package 'bhm' (Bayesian Method)

The R package 'bhm' or biomarker threshold models evaluate the treatment effect, biomarker effect, and treatment by biomarker interaction using hierarchical priors in Bayesian models with MCMC. (An option is available to use profile likelihood with bootstrap, which I did not use.) This method is also able to identify the *optimal* cut point and I used to compare the optimal threshold from the nonparametric bootstrap above:

```
> fit$c.max
56.34997%
   0.3913
```

We see that the two procedures yield similar results for the optimal threshold. Either method can be used for modeling any disease outcomes and statistical models, with the Harrison and Simon R functions providing a very simple and flexible approach via the nonparametric bootstrap method.

11

Cutoff Determination of Continuous Predictive Biomarker Using Group Sequential Methodology

Holmgren [1] has introduced a clever procedure to determine the cutoff (threshold) for a continuous biomarker using the group sequential methodology (GSM). In contrast to the previous approaches discussed in Chapter 10, where we discussed testing for treatment effects, like hazard ratio, in predefined subgroups, this procedure tests the treatment effect in the marker-defined subgroup vs the complement of the subgroup. Holmgren points out there are really four subgroups being considered (treatment vs placebo, marker vs marker-complement). This is a more complex problem to solve than simply testing for a treatment effect in subgroups. For the simpler approach, Jiang et al. [5] discuss a test for biomarker-defined subgroup as well as for detecting a treatment effect in the overall population (if one is present) in the same randomized Phase III trial. But, Holmgren's novel approach enables the marker subgroup and its complement to be tested within the solid framework of GSM methodology of type-I error control while testing several biomarker x treatment hypotheses along the range of biomarker expression values. Since GSM boundaries are readily computed from within R, Holmgren's approach becomes easy to implement for the statistician.

The GSM makes this process extremely easy and preserves the strong control of type I error. In the usual context of GSM, we look at the accumulating subgroups of patients across time in multiple stages. The same concept is applied to the data set where the data is be ordered by marker expression values, instead of time. The precise marker threshold for dichotomizing is unknown or the inflection point for treatment effect along the biomarker range of expression values is unknown.

Holmgren notes that if the objective of the Phase II trial is to see if the drug candidate should proceed to Phase III, with the prior belief that a biomarker could define the effective treatment region, then simply testing the treatment effect in one or more biomarker subgroups is sufficient with adjustment for multiple testing. We discuss this in the previous sections. However, if the objective is to see identify the biomarker expression range, where the magnitude of the treatment effect is maximal, then this approach is very handy. This difference is worth pondering.

11.1 Holmgren's GSM Method for Biomarker Subgroup Selection

Like Holmgren [1], I will discuss the example with a time-to-event outcome; however, this methodology can be easily applied to continuous and count or response data.

Let λ_1, λ_2, λ_3, and λ_4 be the hazard ratios of a time to event, like progression or death in the four subgroups of patients defined by quartiles of the biomarker values (Table 11.1).

This implies the ordering of subjects by marker expression values.

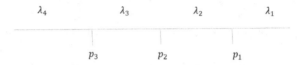

Holmgren gives the formulae for calculating basic probabilities for group sequential stopping boundaries in Table 2 of their paper. The theory is identical to computing Z-statistics for two overlapping groups of subjects corresponding to two analysis times. The methodology is a good match for our context where the subject groups overlap in biomarker percentiles (see the column groupings in Table 1). The calculations are exactly the same and they also extend to continuous, binary response, and time-to-event data.

In order to start using GSM, we also need to choose an alpha spending function. This is one of the advantages of this flexible method because we can spend alpha differentially in each marker subgroup. Holmgren chose the gamma spending function below for illustration, but any method such as the O'Brien and Fleming method could easily be used.

TABLE 11.1

Hazard Ratio and Four Subgroups of Patients Defined by Quartiles of Biomarker Values

Hazard Ratio	Description
λ_1	Treatment effect in subjects whose biomarker expression values are $> p_1$ percentile Example: p_1 = 75th percentile
λ_2	Treatment effect in subjects whose biomarker expression values are between p_1 and p_2 percentile Example: p_2 = 50th percentile
λ_3	Treatment effect in subjects whose biomarker expression values are between p_2 and p_3 percentile Example: p_3 = 25th percentile
λ_4	Treatment effect in subjects whose biomarker expression values are below p_3 percentile Example: p_3 = 25th percentile

11.1.1 Two-Step Procedure

Holmgren defines four hypotheses: H_1, H_2, H_3, and H_4, each of which has several components. H_4 has four components (just like a four-stage interim analysis design); H_3 has three components (like a three-stage interim analysis); and so on. At the end of the trial, say for H_4, we structure the data as if we are carrying out a four-stage interim analysis. Using group sequential boundaries, we test the four components of H_4 with the first analysis being the subjects whose biomarker $> p_1$ and so on. If H_4 rejects, we move on to testing H_3.

If you see the columns of Table 11.2, they are the components of the each hypotheses set and the rows are each of the hypotheses set. For each of the hypotheses set, say H_3, we test the components using GSM (left to right) and then if any component rejects, we move onto H_2. We stop when a hypothesis set fails to reject.

The procedure is thus carried out in two steps:

1. Step 1: Define the hypotheses sets: H_1, H_2, H_3, and H_4, where each will consist of several component tests. GSM is used to test the components of each set.
2. Step 2: Test the hypotheses sets in the order of H_4, H_3, H_2, and H_1. Since they form a closed set of hypothesis, the type I error is preserved when tested in this order.

Why is the second step included? Holmgren [1] shows in Tables 3 and 4 of their paper, by contrasting the tests of H_4 and H_3, that by using the second step, we can use slightly lower Z critical scores to reject the hypotheses in each set than the one before. This makes it easier to reject and find the relevant biomarker region where the treatment effect is greatest.

11.1.2 Strengths and Weaknesses

The strengths of using the two-step Holmgren procedure for GSM are many: (a) power, sample size, and Z-score thresholds for each of the components are easily available in standard software; each component is modeled as an

TABLE 11.2

Hypothesis Testing

Hypotheses	Labels	Biomarker $> p_1$	Biomarker $> p_2$	Biomarker $> p_3$	(All Subjects)
$\lambda_1 = 1, \lambda_2 = 1, \lambda_3 = 1, \lambda_4 = 1$	H_4	X	X	X	X
$\lambda_1 = 1, \lambda_2 = 1, \lambda_3 = 1$	H_3	X	X	X	
$\lambda_1 = 1, \lambda_2 = 1$	H_2	X	X		
$\lambda_1 = 1$	H_1	X			

interim stage in GSM software; (b) flexible alpha spending for biomarker subgroup test; (c) identification of the biomarker region (say between 25th and 50th percentile) where the treatment effect is greatest; and (d) optimally design Phase III study with a clear understanding of hazard ratios in marker subgroup and it's complement and the region where biomarker threshold lies.

The limitation is that a precise threshold value may not be formally identified in the Phase II setting. Holmgren describes an example where H_4, H_3, and H_2 are rejected and H_1 is not. This means we concluded that those with biomarker values greater than the 50th percentile showed a treatment effect. In addition, since H_4 and H_3 also rejected, we can say there was a treatment effect above p_3. What we cannot formally conclude is whether treatment was greater in those above the 50th percentile and those less than the 50th percentile.

Holmgren discusses workaround to this problem. One thing I want to point out is that step 2 is optional. If you have rejections in H_4, then you may have sufficient information regarding which subgroup have activity and can study it further through simulations prior to commencing the Phase III study.

Also note that our example considers equal quartiles of the biomarker; however, this need not be the preferred option in analyzing your data set. You can consider any percentile because it can be represented as an information fraction in the GSM framework.

11.1.3 R Code

The R package 'rpact' [2] was designed and implemented for design, simulation dn analysis of confirmatory adaptive clinical trial designs with continuous, binary, and survival endpoints. I used this package to illustrate the calculations presented in the Holmgren paper. This package is validated for regulatory submissions and is the result of successful collaborations between the founders and several pharmaceutical partners.

Assuming that we are interested in the procedure for testing H_4 hypothesis set, resulting from the gamma (–1) spending function as outlined in the Holmgren paper, we first use the 'rpact' R package to calculate the Z critical scores for testing each of the components. Only one line of code was necessary.

```
>library(rpact)

>ds1=getDesignGroupSequential(informationRates = c(0.25,
0.5,.75,1),sided=1, typeOfDesign = "asHSD",gammaA =
-1,alpha=.1)
>ds1
```

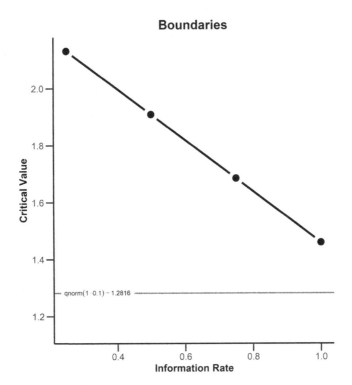

FIGURE 11.1
Critical values for the boundaries vs information rate.

The Z critical scores returned are:
   Output:

```
Cumulative alpha spending: 0.01653, 0.03775, 0.06501, 0.10000
Critical values: 2.131, 1.909, 1.685, 1.460
```

The critical values exactly match those of the Holmgren paper Table 3.
   The plot of the 'ds1' object also shows the boundaries as well (Figure 11.1).

11.2 Sample Size Calculations

One of the extremely useful aspects of the GSM methodology and the R 'rpact' package is the built-in sample size and power calculations. Holmgren calculates the number of events at each 'stage' or biomarker subgroup fraction, alpha spent, and power at each stage. Table 3 of the Holmgren paper shows the sample size and power and type I error under the assumption of detecting a hazard ratio of 0.65 in the study population as a whole. Power was shown to be 80% in the whole population.

Simply, one additional call to a function yields the power, overall and at each stage. Note, the function expects the hazard ratio to be greater than one when favoring the treatment.

```
> p=getPowerSurvival(design = ds1, hazardRatio = 1.54,
maxNumberOfEvents = 106, maxNumberOfSubjects = 250,lambda2=log
(2)/6,directionUpper = TRUE)
> p
```

Design plan parameters and output for survival data:

Design parameters:
  Significance level   : 0.1000
  Test   : one-sided

User defined parameters:
  Lambda (2)   : 0.116
  Hazard ratio   : 1.540
  Maximum number of subjects   : 250.0
  Maximum number of events   : 106.0
  Event time   : 12

Default parameters:
  Type of computation   : Schoenfeld
  Theta H0   : 1
  Direction upper   : TRUE
  Planned allocation ratio   : 1
  Accrual time   : 12
  Piecewise survival times   : 0.00
  Drop-out rate (1)   : 0.000
  Drop-out rate (2)   : 0.000
  Drop-out time   : 12

Sample size and output:
  pi (1)   : 0.882
  pi (2)   : 0.750
  Median (1)   : 3.9
  Median (2)   : 6.0
  Lambda (1)   : 0.178
  Accrual intensity   : 20.8
  Follow up time   : -1.49
  Analysis times [1]   : 4.65
  Analysis times [2]   : 6.91
  Analysis times [3]   : 8.80
  Analysis times [4]   : 10.51
  Expected study duration   : 8.35
  Maximal study duration   : 10.51

```
Number of events by stage [1]                : 26.5
Number of events by stage [2]                : 53.0
Number of events by stage [3]                : 79.5
Number of events by stage [4]                : 106.0
Expected number of events                    : 74.9
Number of subjects [1]                       : 97.0
Number of subjects [2]                       : 144.0
Number of subjects [3]                       : 183.4
Number of subjects [4]                       : 218.9
Expected number of subjects                  : 173.9
Reject per stage [1]                         : 0.154
Reject per stage [2]                         : 0.239
Reject per stage [3]                         : 0.234
Reject per stage [4]                         : 0.175
Overall reject                               : 0.802
Early stop                                   : 0.627
Critical values (effect scale) [1]           : 2.289
Critical values (effect scale) [2]           : 1.689
Critical values (effect scale) [3]           : 1.459
Critical values (effect scale) [4]           : 1.328
Local one-sided significance levels [1]      : 0.01653
Local one-sided significance levels [2]      : 0.02813
Local one-sided significance levels [3]      : 0.04604
Local one-sided significance levels [4]      : 0.07219

Legend:
  (i): values of treatment arm i
  [k]: values at stage k
```

We see that the overall power is 80%; in stage 1 (biomarker > 75th percentile), power is 15.4%; in stage 2 (biomarker > 50th percentile), power is 39.3%; and in stage 3 (biomarker > 25th percentile), power is 62.4%. Therefore, we obtain the exact results of the Holmgren paper.

12

Adaptive Threshold Design

As you can see, it is not essential to know the biomarker cutpoint ahead of Phase II or even Phase III trial commencement. However, not knowing the biomarker or the cutpoint presents statistical challenges that must be overcome. Statistical innovations have paved the way to addressing these challenges in integrating biomarker cutoff finding and testing multiple biomarker subgroups within the hypotheses testing framework for treatment effect in clinical trials. We discussed the Group Sequential Methods (GSM) to explore the cutpoint for biomarker-positive subgroup and testing the subgroup and its complement above in the Holmgren method. The procedure enables exploring several cutpoints in the range of biomarker expression values. This is ideal in the Phase 2 setting of clinical drug development program. This chapter focuses on introducing the adaptive threshold design (ATD) for integrating biomarker threshold selection in Phase 2 or 3 studies. The limitation is that the source code for extensive simulations is not available for download. Nevertheless, here I describe the procedure as laid out by the authors.

The Food and Drug Administration (FDA) is increasingly interested in lending its support for properly designed clinical trials, which used adaptive mechanisms (like GSM and other procedures) to bring the right therapy to patients. The current FDA guidance states: *an adaptive design is defined as a clinical trial design that allows for prospectively planned modifications to one or more aspects of the design based on accumulating data from subjects in the trial* [23].

In this chapter, I will discuss some details about the design proposed by Jiang, Friedlin, and Simon [22], where the procedure for identifying the continuous biomarker threshold and testing biomarker-positive subgroup for treatment effect under type I error rate $\alpha = 0.05$ is developed. Although this ATD does not re-estimate sample size or select new endpoints at the interim of the trial, it is *adaptive* in the sense that it will adaptively identify the subgroup where the treatment effect is maximal. The Holmgren method, using GSM, is similar in its adaptive nature, but is a different procedure.

12.1 The ATD Procedure

The procedure is clearly described in Chapter 14 by Simon [23] as follows:

> As usual, whenever we are engaged in finding an optimal threshold for the biomarker, we are working with a quantitative or

semiquantitative biomarker, and there is evidence that patients with larger values of the biomarker have treatment benefit.

1. The ATD will not be based on the full population, but the overall study-wise type I error rate $\alpha = 0.05$ is controlled for looking at multiple subgroups.

2. The biomarker is assumed to be scaled to have values between [0,1]

3. The null hypothesis at threshold t_i is such that

$$\log(\text{HR}) = c \text{ for } \text{BM} > t_{(i)}$$

$$\begin{cases} = c \text{ for } BM > t_{(i)} \\ 0 \text{ for } BM \le t_{(i)} \end{cases}$$

which means the log hazard ratio is the same for treatment and control groups when biomarker (BM) values are less than or equal to $t_{(i)}$. For larger BM values $> t_i$, the log hazard ratio drops to c (<0). This is a specific shape for the biomarker–treatment interaction, which is a delayed effect.

4. The partial log-likelihoods are maximized with data under each hypothesis (identified by the number of candidate cutpoints). If there are I cutpoints, then a test statistic is computed as $T^* = \max\{L_1, L_2, \ldots, L_I\}$. Note the distribution of the T is not known since if the maximum of several correlated statistics, L_i.

5. The authors derive the null distribution of T^* by permutation. The procedure is permuting the treatment labels and recomputing the likelihood for the permuted data and calculate a new value for T. This is repeated many times. Finally, the significance level is calculated as the proportion of times T exceeds or is equal to T^*. If this global test is rejected at the .05 level, we can conclude there is a biomarker cutpoint above which there is a differential treatment effect for the drug.

6. The last step is identifying which threshold is optimal. This is done by fitting a cutpoint cox proportional hazards model with treatment, biomarker indicator, and a biomarker indicator–treatment interaction terms. One mode is fit for each cutpoint. The P values obtained for the interaction term need to be adjusted by the bootstrap method.

It is also possible to accommodate a quantitative biomarker and establish a treatment effect per one unit increase in the level of biomarker in this procedure.

The power and sample size calculations for this procedure needs simulations of data under various assumptions. The limitation is that the code is not immediately available publicly for use.

13

Adaptive Seamless Design (ASD)

Several authors have proposed adaptive seamless Phase II/III designs. See a comprehensive review of biomarker-guided *nonadaptive* trial designs in the article by Antoniou et al. [8], and a review of *adaptive* biomarker-guided adaptive trial designs in the article by Antoniou et al. [26]. In clinical trials, we can be in complex situation where multiple endpoints (e.g., PFS and OS) are considered in stage I (Phase II) and stage II (Phase III) trials, as well as uncertainty exists with respect to which population (biomarker positive (BM+) or all subjects) to study. Here, I assume that the biomarker threshold is known and the subjects can be accurately separated into two groups with one group (BM+) likely to respond more than the biomarker-negative subgroup. Jenkins, Stone, and Jennison [27] present this correlated time-to-event data endpoints design where PFS is used for stage I and OS for stage II; where the BM+ subgroup and overall populations can be both tested with co-primary endpoints in a single seamless confirmatory trial. One of the main advantages of this design is that patients from both stages I and II contribute to the calculation of the test statistics for OS, the final endpoint for approval. This is why this design saves time and cost compared to running two separate trials. The second advantage is subpopulation selection that is included in this design (if the overall population does not have a viable treatment effect signal). The third advantage is that we can use different but correlated endpoints for testing the efficacies of stages I and II.

13.1 ASD: A Two-Stage Design

This type of design is sometimes also called *adaptive enrichment* designs. In this specific case, it is a two-stage design, where in a first stage patients are recruited from the full population. Then, in an interim analysis, based on interim data at the end of the first stage, the trial design of the second stage may be adapted to patients in the BM+ subgroup. No break is observed between learning (stage I) and confirming (stage II). None of the information gained in stage I is lost in the final analysis; hence, the design is *inferentially* seamless, as well as *operationally* seamless.

At the interim analysis, the authors consider an intermediate time-to-event endpoint, PFS, and the trial can either

- continue in co-primary populations ∀ (all-comers) and *BM+* subgroup
- continue in *BM+* subgroup only
- continue in the full population ∀ without an analysis in *BM+* subgroup
- stop for futility

The stage I patients remain in the trial and continue to be monitored for survival events for a prespecified follow-up time (not to be modified at interim analysis). Meanwhile, more subjects are newly recruited to stage II. Information on the final time-to-event endpoint, OS, can be combined from subjects of both stages. The read-out from this analysis will be at the end of the trial.

The design described by Jennison [27] is shown in Figure 13.1.

The decision rule is illustrated in Table 13.1.

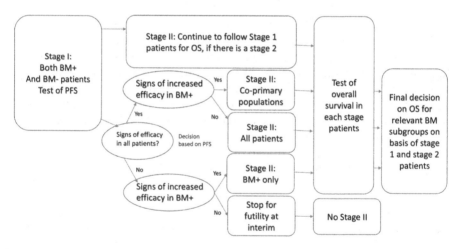

FIGURE 13.1
Seamless, adaptive Phase II–III design.

TABLE 13.1

Decision Rule

PFS Hazard Ratio Estimates at the Interim Analysis	$\widehat{HR}^{\lor} < 0.8$	$\widehat{HR}^{\lor} \geq 0.8$
$\widehat{HR}^{BM+} < 0.6$	Continue with co-primary analysis	Continue in subgroup *BM* + only
$\widehat{HR}^{BM+} \geq 0.6$	Continue in all-comers ∀ only	Stop for futility

13.2 ASD: Controlling Type I Error

The authors use numerous statistical methods to control the studywise Type I error of 0.05, which they explain in their paper. They consider both all-comers ∀ and the subpopulation *BM+* separately for multiple one-sided hypothesis tests about the treatment effect. Within each population, there is a single null hypothesis of no difference in overall survival between treatment and control. Using the closure principle, a null hypothesis in either population can be rejected if all intersection hypotheses that imply the null are also rejected. They adjust the *P* values from the all-comers and biomarker subgroup using the Hochberg correction procedure.

At the end of the study, they combine the *P* values from both stages in the final analysis on all subjects in the relevant population, using an inverse-normal combination test with weights w_{St_I} and w_{St_II} such that $w_{St\_I}^2 + w_{St\_II}^2 = 1$. They recommend the weights w_1 and w_2 be chosen to be proportional to the square roots of the numbers of overall survival events observed during each stage. Refer to the paper to see which hypotheses will need to be tested in the final analysis depending on which population is selected.

13.3 R Package 'asd'

Parsons [28] has given a very useful simulation tool in the R package 'asd' for the Jenkins adaptive seamless stage I/stage II design for oncology trials using correlated survival endpoints. I reproduce the biomarker subgroup selection example written in the package primer by Parsons et al. [29] here.

Operational characteristics of this type of design is implemented in a single R command of the subpop.sim() function with the appropriate design parameters.

The notation used in the Parsons paper [28] in sections 2 and 3 may be useful to the reader to understand the assumptions, as well as extend the models behind the simulations. For this example, the authors assume both PFS and OS hazard ratios to be 0.6 in the subgroup *BM+* and 0.9 in ∀ all-comers. The correlation between endpoints is 0.5.

13.4 Example and R Code

Let us set the stage I sample size to 125 patients per arm and the stage II sample size to 250 patients per arm if we progress to all-comers in the full population and to 200 patients per arm if we progress in the subgroup only.

The *BM+* subgroup prevalence is fixed at 0.3. The authors use the futility rule for selection at interim, with limits for the subgroup and full population both set to 0, this scenario can be implemented using the following R function call in the package:

```
out=subpop.sim(n=list(stage1=125,enrich=200,stage2=250),
effect=
list(early=c(0.6,0.9),final=c(0.6,0.9)),
sprev=0.3,outcome=list(early="T",final="T"),
nsim=10000,corr=0.5,seed=617,select="futility",
selim=c(0,0),level=0.025,method="CT-SD")
```

The 'method = CT-SD' option implements the combination test method with Spiessens and Debois' testing procedure [30].

```
hypotheses rejected and group selection options at stage 1 (n):
          Hs        Hf     Hs+Hf      Hs+f         n        n%
sub     2171         0         0      2172      2238     22.38
full       0        28         0        34       156      1.56
both    5237      1740      1714      5288      7230     72.30
total   7408      1768      1714      7494      9624         -
%      74.08     17.68     17.14     74.94     96.24         -
reject Hs and/or Hf =   74.62%
```

The output shows that in 74%, 18%, and 17% of the simulations in the subgroup, full population, and both, the null hypothesis is rejected, respectively. The final two columns give a breakdown of the selections made at the interim analysis; 22% of the simulations were continued in the subgroup only; 2% in the full population only, 72% in both, and 4% (100 − (22.38 + 1.56 + 72.3)) were stopped for futility. The user may run the above code for a grid of futility rule limits. Further discussions on simulating the trial are available in the primer.

References

1. Holmgren E. (2017). The application of group sequential stopping boundaries to evaluate the treatment effect of an experimental agent across a range of biomarker expression. *Contemp. Clin. Trials*, 63:13–18.
2. Wassmer G, Pahlke F. (2019). rpact: Confirmatory Adaptive Clinical Trial Design and Analysis. R package version 2.0.2. https://CRAN.R-project.org/package=rpact
3. Glimm E, Di Scala L. (2015). An approach to confirmatory testing of subpopulations in clinical trials. *Biom. J.*, 57:897–913. doi:10.1002/bimj.201400006.

4. Freidlin B, Sun Z, Gray R, Korn EL. (2013). Phase III clinical trials that integrate treatment and biomarker evaluation. *J Clin. Oncol.*, 31:3158–3161.
5. Halabi S, Michiels S. (2019). *Textbook of Clinical Trials in Oncology: A Statistical Perspective*. Boca Raton, FL: CRC Press.
6. Dmitrienko A, Tamhane AC, Bretz F. (2010). *Multiple Testing Problems in Pharmaceutical Statistics*. Boca Raton, FL: Chapman & Hall/CRC.
7. https://www.cytel.com/hubfs/0-library-0/pdfs/SiZ-MCP-Webinar-10-4-2011-new.pdf
8. Antoniou M, Kolamunnage-Dona R, Jorgensen AL. (2017). Biomarker-guided non-adaptive trial designs in phase II and phase III: A methodological review. *J. Pers. Med.*, 7:1.
9. Shak S. (1999). Overview of the trastuzumab(Herceptin) anti-HER2 monoclonal antibody clinical program in HER2-overexpressing metastatic breast cancer. Herceptin multinational investigator study group. *Semin. Oncol.*,26:71–77.
10. Chapman PB, Hauschild A, Robert C et al. (2011). Improved survival with vemurafenib in melanoma with BRAF V600E mutation. *N. Engl. J. Med.*, 364:2507–2516.
11. Haller B, Ulm K, Hapfelmeier A. (2019). A simulation study comparing different statistical approaches for the identification of predictive biomarkers. *Comput. Math. Methods Med.*, 7037230. doi:10.1155/2019/7037230.
12. Hothorn T, Lausen B. (2003). On the exact distribution of maximally selected rank statistics. *Comput. Stat. Data Anal.*, 43(2):121–137. doi:10.1016/S0167-9473(02)00225.
13. Bonetti M, Gelber RD. (2000). A graphical method to assess treatment-covariate interactions using the Cox model on subsets of the data. *Stat. Med.*, 19(19):2595–2609.
14. Yip WK. with contributions from Ann Lazar, David Zahrieh, Chip Cole, Ann Lazar, Marco Bonetti, Victoria Wang, William Barcella and Richard Gelber (2018). stepp: Subpopulation Treatment Effect Pattern Plot (STEPP). R package version 3.2.0.0. https://CRAN.R-project.org/package=stepp
15. Hothorn T. (2017). maxstat: Maximally Selected Rank Statistics. R package version 0.7-25. https://CRAN.R-project.org/package=maxstat
16. Morrison J, Simon N. Rank conditional coverage and confidence intervals in high dimensional problems, ArXiv e-prints [arXiv:1702.06986].
17. Chen B. (2017). _A Package for Biomarker Threshold Models_. R package version 1.15. https://CRAN.R-project.org/package=bhm
18. Chen B, Jiang W, Tu D. (2014). A hierarchical bayes model for biomarker subset effects in clinical trials. *Comput. Stat. Data Anal.*, 71:324–334.
19. Fang T, Mackillop W, Jiang W, Hildesheim A, Wacholder S, Chen B. (2017). A Bayesian method for risk window estimation with application to HPV vaccine trial. *Comput. Stat. Data Anal.*, 112:53–62.
20. Morrison J. (2019). *Treatment Effects in Nested Subgroups (Section 3.2)*. Jean997.github.io. https://jean997.github.io/rccSims/biomarker_sims.html#session_information
21. Buyse M, Michiels S, Sargent DJ, Grothey A, Matheson A, de Gramont A. (2011). Integrating biomarkers in clinical trials. *Expert Rev. Mol. Diagn.*, 11:2, 171–182. doi:10.1586/erm.10.120.
22. Jiang W., Freidlin B, Simon R. (2007). Biomarker-adaptive threshold design: A procedure for evaluating treatment with possible biomarker-defined subset effect. *JNCI: J. Natl. Cancer Inst.*, 99(13):1036–1043. doi:10.1093/jnci/djm022.

23. FDA, Adaptive design for clinical trials for drugs and biologics, Draft Guidance (2018) https://www.fda.gov/media/78495/download

24. Jørgensen JT. (2019) *Companion and Complementary Diagnostics: From Biomarker Discovery to Clinical Implementation.* 1st edition. Elsevier Science. https://www.fda.gov/media/81309/download

25. Benjamini Y, Hochberg Y. (1995). *J R. Stat. Soc. Series B (Methodological).*, 57(1):289–300.

26. Antoniou M, Jorgensen AL, Kolamunnage-Dona R. (2016). Biomarker-guided adaptive trial designs in phase II and phase III: A methodological review. *PLoS One*, 11:e0149803. doi:10.1371/journal.pone.0149803.

27. Jenkins M, Stone A, Jennison C. (2011). An adaptive seamless phase II/III design for oncology trials with subpopulation selection using correlated survival endpoint. *Pharmaceut. Statist.*, 10(4). 347–356. doi:10.1002/pst.472.

28. Parsons N. (2016). asd: Simulations for Adaptive Seamless Designs. R package version 2.2. https://CRAN.R-project.org/package=asd

29. Parsons N, Friede T, Todd S, Stallard N. (2011). Software tools for implementing simulation studies in adaptive seamless designs: Introducing R package ASD. *Trials*, 12(Suppl 1):A8. doi:10.1186/1745-6215-12-S1-A8.

30. Spiessens B, Debois M. (2010). Adjusted significance levels for subgroup analysis in clinical trials. *Contemp. Clin. Trials*, 31:647–656.

31. Olsen D, Jørgensen J. (2014). Companion diagnostics for targeted cancer drugs—Clinical and regulatory aspects. *Front. Oncol.*, 4:105. doi:10.3389/fonc.2014.00105.

32. Draft Guidance for Industry, Clinical Laboratories, and FDA Staff In Vitro Diagnostic Multivariate Index Assays. https://www.fda.gov/media/81309/download

33. US Food and Drug Administration. Draft Guidance for Industry and Food and Drug Administration Staff – In vitro Companion Diagnostic D https://www.fda.gov/media/81309/download

34. US Food and Drug Administration. Draft Guidance for Industry and Food and Drug Administration Staff – In vitro Companion Diagnostic Device.

Section III

Surrogate Endpoints

14

Introduction

In clinical trials, a surrogate endpoint measures the effect of a specific treatment that may show good correlation with the effect measured by an approved and acceptable clinical endpoint [1]. The surrogate endpoint, which is a biomarker, measured in the patient in the clinical trial, does not have to measure the clinical benefit directly – but it should be able to predict the clinical benefit. The National Institutes of Health (USA) defines surrogate endpoint as 'a biomarker intended to substitute for a clinical endpoint'. According to the NCI (National Cancer Institute) [2], using surrogate endpoints in clinical trials may allow earlier approval of new drugs in serious illnesses, like cancer. The problem is that statistical and clinical burden of proof remains high, since surrogate endpoints are not always true indicators or nor do they capture the full treatment effect.

A clinical trial can use either the real, objective endpoint or an approved surrogate endpoint in the study. The clinical endpoint represents direct clinical benefit such as survival. Survival (OS) is a direct benefit that may take years to measure in cancer trials, for example. As treatments improve with science, newer treatments may face a staggering uphill climb to prove the efficacy on the scale of a true clinical benefit, like OS. In recent trials reported in ASCO 2017 [3] on HER2-positive breast cancer, the median follow-up times reported were between three years and ten years. In general, for breast cancer trials, the follow-up time can be short (0–5 years), moderate (5–10 years), or long (10–20 years). A patient sometimes consents to being blinded to the treatment for more than 10 years while being treated for her disease. Not only is it challenging to conduct a trial where the primary clinical endpoints take a long time to measure (early stage of cancer progression, for example) but also, in later stage of cancer progression, the underlying effect of treatment on the true endpoint is obscured by many lines of treatment. While the longer-term studies may provide valuable insight into disease progression, recurrence, and remission in some settings, it is not always feasible or useful to wait to measure those endpoints for every drug and/or in every disease setting. Even if the drug manufacturer waited, the new treatment may not be relevant by the time it is approved because newer treatment options may well be available for patients. For many such reasons, trialists look for surrogate endpoints instead to predict clinical benefit.

In oncology trials, for example, tumor shrinkage can be shown to predict longer survival in clinical trials for drugs intended to treat some cancers. So, response rates defined from tumor shrinkage have been used as surrogate for overall survival in some approvals for cancer treatment. Clinicians often grapple with the questions, which biomarkers can be used as surrogate to predict true clinical endpoints? The answer depends on where we are in the process of validating the surrogate endpoint in that disease indication. While some surrogate endpoints are already validated or more established in a particular disease area and treatment context, others are seen as reasonably likely to predict clinical benefit. Using this latter type of surrogate is the basis of accelerated approval from the Food and Drug Administration (FDA). This type of approval on the intermediate (surrogate) endpoint is conditional upon showing a statistically significant treatment effect on the primary clinical (true) endpoint by continuing to follow the patients' progress under the treatments.

The FDA [3a] categorizes surrogate endpoints in roughly three hierarchical categories:

- candidate surrogate endpoint
- reasonably likely surrogate endpoint
- validated surrogate endpoint

The top category is the least accepted and the bottom the most accepted. The validated surrogate is established for a specific disease, patient population, and class of drugs. However, the candidate surrogate endpoint is a correlated to the clinical endpoint and is a measure of biological activity (since it is a biomarker), but it is not yet established at a more rigorous level. We will discuss the necessary requirements further below.

The area of validating biomarkers as surrogate endpoints is an active area of research in the FDA. Consequently, more and more biomarkers are being qualified with the advancement of our understanding of their role in the disease and the therapeutic intervention process on the disease. Between 2010 and 2012, the FDA approved 45% of new drugs based on surrogate endpoint. When the surrogate endpoint has been validated, the approval type is regular for a trial using that surrogate endpoint in that disease area. When the biomarker is shown as a surrogate endpoint, which is 'reasonably likely to predict the clinical benefit', the approval type is accelerated with full approval conditional on data being available from the true clinical endpoint. The accelerated approval allows a more expedient access to the new treatment to patients. When the biomarker is a novel candidate for a clinical endpoint, a type C meeting is recommended between the sponsor and the FDA in the preliminary stages of clinical development for appropriate strategy.

14.1 Examples of Surrogate Endpoints

Up until an endpoint is known as an established surrogate endpoint in a disease area, it is still considered a biomarker. Here, we do not refer to a predictive biomarker, which is measured prior to the start of treatment but to one that is measured after treatment has begun.

A few common surrogate endpoints for clinical trials of cancer treatments are [4] as follows:

- Time to Progression (TTP): The length of time from the date of diagnosis or the start of treatment for a disease until the disease starts to get worse or spread to other parts of the body.
- Progression-Free Survival: The length of time between treatment and measurable worsening of the disease. Generally, it is used to study advanced diseases that are unlikely to be removed entirely.
- Response Rate (RR): The percentage of patients whose cancer shrinks or disappears after treatment.

And the true clinical benefit for many cancers is overall survival (OS) over the time between treatment initiation and death. This measure includes death from any cause, including both the disease being treated and unrelated conditions. This means that OS, unlike some other endpoints, measures both the impact of a treatment after relapse and the survival impact of treatment side effects.

A list of currently approved surrogate endpoints for all adult and pediatric disease areas is available at the FDA website [3b]. The latest one is dated July 23, 2018, and it is updated every six months.

Surrogate endpoints listed at the FDA are established in specific types of disease areas, patient population, and drug mechanism of action. Sometimes a surrogate endpoint may have some limitations in some context, for example, response rate may not translate to overall survival if there is severe toxicity of the drug, that is why the list is specific to disease, patient population, and MOA (mechanism of action of the drug).

For reader's interest, we show the surrogates mentioned for hematological malignancies [3c] in adults in Table 14.1.

Of course, there are surrogate endpoints in other disease areas besides cancer, for example, CD4 cell count change as a surrogate for time to progression to AIDS or death. We will cover this example later.

TABLE 14.1

List of Surrogate Endpoints for hematological malignancies

Disease or Use	Patient Population	Surrogate Endpoint	Type of Approval Appropriate for	Drug Mechanism of Action
Cancer: hematological malignancies	Patients with diffuse large B-cell lymphoma	Event-free survival (EFS)[c]	Traditional	Mechanism agnostic[a]
Cancer: hematological malignancies	Patients with chronic myeloid leukemia; hypereosinophilic syndrome/chronic eosinophilic leukemia	Major hematologic response	Accelerated/ Traditional[b]	Mechanism agnostic[a]
Cancer: hematological malignancies	Patients with acute myeloid leukemia and acute lymphoblastic leukemia	Durable complete remission rate	Accelerated/ Traditional[b]	Mechanism agnostic[a]
Cancer: hematological malignancies	Patients with acute lymphoblastic leukemia; myelodysplastic/ myeloproliferative diseases; chronic myeloid leukemia	Major hematologic response and cytogenic response	Accelerated/ Traditional[b]	Mechanism agnostic[a]
Cancer: hematological malignancies	Patients with B-cell precursor acute lymphoblastic leukemia in first or second complete remission	Minimal residual disease response rate	Accelerated	Mechanism agnostic[a]
Cancer: hematological malignancies	Patients with T-cell lymphoma; mantle cell lymphoma; classical Hodgkin lymphoma; anaplastic large cell lymphoma and mycosis fungoides; non-Hodgkin's lymphoma; multiple myeloma; chronic myeloid leukemia; acute lymphoblastic leukemia; small lymphocytic lymphoma; Waldenström's macroglobulinemia; marginal zone lymphoma	Durable objective overall response rate (ORR)	Accelerated/ Traditional[b]	Mechanism agnostic[a]

(Continued)

TABLE 14.1 (*Continued*)

List of Surrogate Endpoints for hematological malignancies

Disease or Use	Patient Population	Surrogate Endpoint	Type of Approval Appropriate for	Drug Mechanism of Action
Cancer: hematological malignancies	Patients with multiple myeloma; mantle cell lymphoma; classical Hodgkin lymphoma; follicular lymphoma; diffuse large B-cell lymphoma; chronic myeloid leukemia; chronic lymphocytic leukemia; cutaneous T-cell lymphoma; all other non-Hodgkin lymphoma	Progression-Free Survival	Traditional	Mechanism agnostic[a]

[a] Mechanism agnostic refers to cases where there are many mechanisms of action associated with a surrogate endpoint, so it is not directly related to a particular causal pathway.

[b] Endpoints based on changes in tumor burden may be used for both traditional and accelerated approval depending on context of use, including factors such as disease, effect size, effect duration, residual uncertainty, and benefits of other available therapy.

[c] The agency anticipates that this surrogate endpoint could be appropriate for use as a primary efficacy clinical trial endpoint for drug or biological approval, although it has not yet been used to support an approved NDA or BLA.

14.2 All Pharmacodynamic Biomarkers Are Not Surrogate Endpoints

Yes, that is right! A biomarker can have utility as a pharmacodynamic bio-marker but not necessarily meet the more stringent requirements to be a surrogate endpoint. A biomarker needs to be in the disease causal pathway as well as be modulated by treatment. Many initial studies tend to overesti-mate the treatment effect captured by the surrogate biomarker. An indepen-dent data set is required to verify the surrogacy hypotheses. Fleming and DeMets [21] give this clear graphic, which exemplify five scenarios where a biomarker could be considered as surrogate:

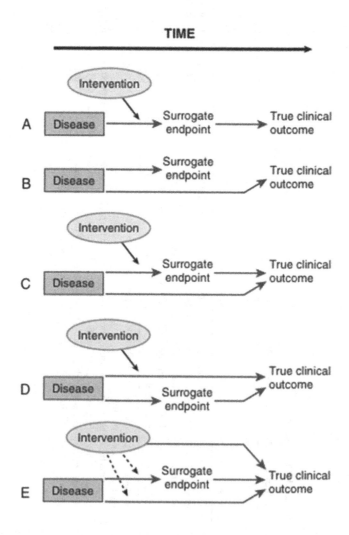

- Scenario A: ideal scenario for the biomarker to be a surrogate endpoint
- Scenario B: biomarker is not in the disease causal pathway
- Scenario C: multiple causal pathways for disease
- Scenario D: biomarker does not capture treatment effect
- Scenario E: treatment affects clinical outcome outside of disease mechanism

The dotted lines are possible mechanisms of action. As you can see biomarkers serve many purpose but the burden for proving such a biomarker is a surrogate endpoint is high.

14.3 Establishing Surrogacy: Prentice Criteria

There are two types of use for surrogate endpoints:

- Prognostic: Here, the surrogate endpoint is associated with the clinical endpoint but possibly observed earlier. For example, tumor response as a surrogate for the OS either within the same trial or the prognostic endpoint is measured in earlier phase trials and gives a hint of clinical endpoint to be measured in later phase trials.
- Predictive: Here, the surrogate endpoint must also capture the treatment effect on the clinical endpoint.

So, the intuition behind a biomarker that acts as a surrogate endpoint (S) for the true endpoint (T) is that there has to be a strong correlation of association between S and T; it is correct only partially. In other words, correlation is a necessary but not sufficient condition to establish surrogacy.

Prentice [6] formally defined what a surrogate endpoint is in statistical terms. Prentice's criteria consist of four components that would qualify a biomarker as a fully validated surrogate endpoint. Suppose Z is the treatment indicator, surrogate is S, and the true endpoint is T, then:

$$f(S\,|\,Z) \neq f(S)$$

$$f(T\,|\,Z) \neq f(T)$$

$$f(T\,|\,S) \neq f(T)$$

$$f(T\,|\,S,Z) = f(T\,|\,S)$$

These components mean that treatment has an effect on both surrogate and true endpoints, the surrogate endpoint has a significant effect on the true endpoint, and the full effect of treatment is captured by the effect of the surrogate on the treatment. The first two associations can be shown in the context of randomized trials. The very first association requires conducting smaller trials typically relative to the larger ones required to establish the second association. The third association can be established both within a trial or across trials (prognostic studies).

The last criterion is very appealing, but quite stringent. It would not qualify a surrogate, which only partially explains the effect of the treatment on the true endpoint.

However, taken together the Prentice criteria establish both the correlation and the capture parts of the surrogacy requirements. The Prentice criteria imply that $Z \to S \to T$ which is a Markov Chain. Hence, in addition to the statistical tests, the surrogate endpoint is shown to be mechanistically linked to the disease–drug mechanism of action as well.

In this section, it behooves to provide an example of the single trial with normally distributed surrogate (S_j) and real (T_j) endpoints for subject j. The following four models would be used to evaluate the Prentice criteria:

- $S_j = \mu_S + \alpha Z_j + \epsilon_{S_j}$
- $T_j = \mu_T + \beta Z_j + \epsilon_{T_j}$
- $T_j = \mu + \gamma S_j + \epsilon_j$
- $T_j = \mu + \beta_S Z_j + \gamma S_j + \varepsilon$

where ϵ_{S_j} and ϵ_{T_j} are multivariate normal with mean zero and covariance matrix

$$\Sigma = \begin{matrix} \sigma_{SS} & \sigma_{ST} \\ & \sigma_{TT} \end{matrix}$$

Examples of other distributions are given by Molenberghs et al. [6d] and are available in the wide literature on surrogate endpoints.

14.3.1 Proportion of Treatment Effect Explained by the Surrogate

Freedman et al. [6a] proposed to estimate the proportion of treatment explained by the surrogate as $PTE = 1 - \frac{\beta_S}{\beta}$, where β_S and β are the treatment effects of the surrogate and clinical endpoints, respectively, from the models f(T|S, Z) and f(T|Z), respectively. Freedman introduced this quantity as a way of not having to test the equality of the 4th Prentice criterion, but instead achieve the same result by estimating PE. It was assumed that PE greater than a threshold 0.75 would be considered useful for establishing surrogacy. So, the lower limit of the 95%CI of PTE would need to lie above the threshold.

However, this estimate has some criticism, since PTE is not constrained in the unit (0,1) and also shows high variability in practice [6b], resulting in wide confidence intervals. Alternatively, the Prentice and Freedman approaches, proposed as single trial level statistics, as well as other practical approaches encompassing multiple trials were proposed later.

14.4 Meta-analytic Framework

Meta-analyses of several randomized clinical trials have been widely used for the validation of surrogate endpoints [6c]. The idea is to combine the data from multiple trials and then regress the observed treatment effect for the clinical endpoint on the observed treatment effect as measured by the surrogate. Of course, quantifying the treatment effect on a single endpoint is not the objective here.

Quantifying surrogacy between endpoints has two requirements:

- Requirement #1: Trial level – Assess the ability of the treatment effect of the surrogate endpoint to predict the true endpoint (R^2_{trial})
- Requirement #2: Individual level – Assess the correlation between the surrogate and true endpoints after adjusting for treatment (R^2_{indiv})

Therefore, establishing surrogacy is achieved in two stages, one for each of the above requirements. Statistical models are used in both stages to (a) predict the treatment effect on the true endpoint from the treatment effect captured by the surrogate, and (b) establish high correlation between the two endpoints.

The meta-analytic regression framework is used to assess the trial-level or summary-level surrogacy across trials.

It would be unrealistic to expect $R^2_{trial} = 1$, since that would indicate a perfect surrogate; instead a realistic approach would be to get an estimate which points to a reliable and robust surrogate for the true clinical endpoint. In the next chapter we will discuss the meta-analytic framework in more details and provide the R code for the analysis for specific endpoints used in the oncology for Requirement #1.

15

Requirement # 1: Trial Level – Correlation
Between Hazard Ratios in Progression-Free
Survival and Overall Survival Across Trials

Let us consider the example of solid tumors in oncology. In this setting, much work has been done over the past decade using meta-analytic techniques to investigate progression-related endpoints as possible surrogates for overall survival (OS) in patients [8–12]. Here, the objective is to establish the relationships between the treatment effects along each endpoint, rather than to summarize the treatment effect on a single endpoint. For example, based on summary data from multiple clinical trials, the hazard ratios (HRs) for comparing two treatments on OS (HR^{os}) can be regressed on the HRs of treatment groups for progression-free survival (HR^{pfs}). The logarithmic transformation is typically used in this context and a linear regression model with an equation such as the following is implemented:

$$\log\left(HR^{os}{}_i\right) = \mu + \left(\beta \times \log\left(HR^{pfs}{}_i\right)\right) + \varepsilon_i \tag{15.1}$$

where μ represents an intercept, β is the slope of the linear relationship of the HRs, and ε is the residual variance. In Equation (15.1), each study (i) contributes one observation, typically weighted by the number of subjects in the ITT or the variance of the study-specific HR. Such an analysis expresses the relationship between differences in effect sizes for progression and survival across multiple trials and gives an idea of how strongly the treatment effects on each endpoint are associated with each other under the assumption of a linear relationship.

In other words, the meta-regression equation shows the predicted relationship between the HRs for progression-free survival (PFS) and OS, based on the studies included.

15.1 Meta-Analytic Regression

If the slope (β) of the equation above equals 1, and the intercept is minimal, the treatment effects on survival are expected to be of similar magnitude to effects on PFS. The intercept being close to 0 means that no treatment effect on PFS predicts there would be no treatment effect on OS. Models may address covariates or factors that can influence the endpoint relationship, and sometimes the meta-analysis is repeated on different patient subgroups or risk groups or subsets of studies.

Meta-analytic regression equations take many different forms in the published literature, depending which endpoints are evaluated, whether transformations (like logarithms for hazard or odds ratios) are needed, what is the most appropriate statistical model to be implemented, and how weights for each study are to be calculated [14].

There are several metrics for presenting the strength of the trial-level surrogacy:

- The simple correlation r is between the treatment effect measures across trials. Correlation values are close to 1 if the treatment effects tend to go in the same direction. In other words, correlation is high if the HRs for PFS and OS are similar across trials; correlation is low if the HRs are unrelated or in opposite directions.

- The R^2_{trial} is derived from the meta-regression equation to indicate how much variance in log(OS) is explained by the potential surrogate log(PFS). In the very simplest case, where they are no other covariates, R^2 is equal to a squared correlation estimate (i.e., $R^2 = r \times r$). R^2_{trial} addresses whether treatment effects on the surrogate endpoint are associated with treatment effects on survival, it is particularly important for drug development.

R^2_{trial} values below 0.33 are considered weak evidence; values between 0.33 and 0.67 indicate moderate and above 0.67 denote strong evidence of surrogacy at trial levels.

- The slope β of the regression equation
- The mean square error (MSE) of the regression
- The mean square prediction error (MSPE) from leave one out cross-validation of the regression model

Lastly, there is a drawback in the meta-analysis framework for summarizing the data by a single treatment effect per trial, which is ecological correlation or bias, where grouped data tend to show stronger correlation than individual data for a pair of variables. There are two points I want to make here. First, you may be interested in grouped data (trial level) as well as individual level (within trial) to estimate the correlation between the clinical endpoint and the surrogate. In this case, it is fine to characterize the correlation at both levels. Second, there are multiple ways of correcting for bias arising out of grouped data, for example, one such procedure is to use the inverse of variance of the estimated slope β as weights in linear regression.

Note that we could also model the relationship between a binary endpoint (S) and a survival endpoint (T) by following the same modeling approach for log (odds ratio) and log (HR).

15.2 Example of R Code in Mesothelioma Data

The analysis for validation of PFS as a surrogate endpoint for OS in malignant mesothelioma was presented in a paper by Wang et al. [13]. The data sets consisted of single arm trials and HRs were constructed comparing risk groups.

We use this data set as an example here and present the R code for analysis.

The Weighted Least Square (WLS) model was fit to the Mesothelioma Data for the EORTC Risk Group (Poor, Good Prognosis). The data is given in the Supplemental Appendices Figure B1 in Wang et al., 'The Oncologist 2017'.

Note, I am using the sample size of trial as weights in the linear regression code below; however, as mentioned earlier, you could also use the inverse of the variance of the estimated trial-level slope β parameter as weights if you want to infer individual-level correlation from trial-level data.

Step 1. Read in Data

The R code for reading data is shown below.

```
PFSHR=c(1.45,.95,1.51,1.78,.81,2.09,1.21,1.69,1.13,1.26,1.75,
2.19,2.87,1.52,.92,2.07,1.28)
n=c(33,34,41,44,50,35,20,39,32,17,28,42,45,49,42,23,33)
HR=c(1.77,.99,1.52,1.74,1.12,3.53,1.86,1.84,2.12,1.65,3.44,
2.74,1.23,1.8,1.13,2.01,1.91)
```

Step 2. WLS model fit

The following R code illustrates how to get the WLS model results using log(HR-PFS) to predict the log(HR-OS) for EORTC Risk Group (Poor, Good Prognosis) in Table 4 in the paper for the first row.

```
library(knitr); library(pander)
M=lm(log(HR)~log(PFSHR),weights=n)
R_squared = round(summary(M)$r.squared,2)
pander(M)
```

Fitting linear model: log(HR) ~ log(PFSHR)

	Estimate	Std. Error	t value	Pr(>|t|)
(Intercept)	0.3523	0.118	2.985	0.009254
log(PFSHR)	0.5137	0.2244	2.29	0.03696

Following Equation 15.1 from above, the specific equation for this data set would be:

$$\log(\mathrm{HR}_i^{os}) = 0.35 + (.51 \times \log(\mathrm{HR}_i^{pfs})) + \varepsilon_i \qquad (15.2)$$

This denotes that there is a 49% lower risk on OS associated with the poor prognosis EWORTC group compared to the risk on PFS. The authors of the paper evaluated the shrinkage or attenuation of PFS surrogacy of 49% for OS further with the leave-one-out-cross-validation (LOOCV) tool. We provide the code below.

Step 3. Extract MSPE (mean square prediction error)

```
library(DAAG)
## Loading required package: lattice
RISK=data.frame(n,HR,PFSHR,lHR=log(HR),lPFSHR=log(PFSHR))
cv = CVlm(data=RISK,form.lm=formula(lHR~lPFSHR,weights=n),
m=nrow(RISK), seed=617, plotit = FALSE)
MSPE = attr(cv, "ms")
```

Step 4. Extract MSE (mean square error)

```
library(ISLR); library(modelr);library(purrr)
loocv.data=crossv_kfold(RISK,k=nrow(RISK))
loocv.models=map(loocv.data$train,~lm(lHR~lPFSHR,weights=n,
data=RISK ))
loocv.mse=map2_dbl(loocv.models,loocv.data$test,mse)
MSE=mean(loocv.mse)

WLS_stats = data.frame(R_squared = round(summary(M)$r.
squared,2),
          MSPE = round(attr(cv, "ms"),2),
          MSE = round(MSE,2))
knitr::kable(WLS_stats, caption = "WLS model statistics.",
floating.environment="sidewaystable")
```

WLS model statistics

R_squared	MSPE	MSE
0.26	0.14	0.09

We see that R^2_{trial} is weak, since only 26% of the variability in log(OS) is explained by the linear regression on log(PFS). The MSPE and MSE are low, and the MSPE is larger than MSE. This makes sense because we expect the prediction error to be higher than the error from fitting all the data points. The authors concluded that the results could not support the surrogacy and further investigation was needed to establish surrogacy.

Step 5. WLS regression Plot

The following plot was from WLS regression of OS log HR on PFS log HR across all trials with the sample sizes as weights (Figure 15.1).

```
plot(x=log(PFSHR), y=log(HR), xlim=c(-1,2), ylim=c(-1,2),
type="n",
    main="WLS regression across all trials\n EORTC Risk
    Group",
    xlab="PFS log HR", ylab = "OS log HR")
points(x=log(PFSHR), y=log(HR), cex=n/min(n, na.rm=T),
col="blue")
abline(M$coefficients, lwd=1.8)
legend("top", paste("WLS R Square = ", round(summary(M)$r.
squared,2)), bty="n")
```

This figure matches Figure 2 of the mesothelioma data set [13] for the first panel, which plots the weighted least squares (WLS) regression line in the EORTC risk groups through the summary-level HRs and weighted with the size of the trial.

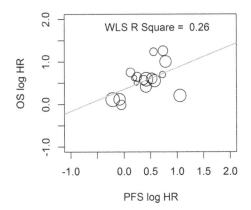

FIGURE 15.1
Meta-Analysis for showing surrogacy PFS and OS.

16

Requirement # 2: Individual Level – Assess the Correlation Between the Surrogate and True Endpoints After Adjusting for Treatment (R^2_{indiv})

Surrogate endpoints are preferred often because of the convenience of measuring them over the true endpoint in clinical trials. When trial data is available, R^2_{trial} denotes the trial-level surrogacy (requirement #1) and R^2_{indiv} (or Kendals τ) denotes the individual-level surrogacy (requirement #2). You might think establishing a correlation between the two endpoints measured on individuals within a trial is matter of performing a simple regression. However, when we model the relationship as a paired variable (bivariate random variable), the process is more precise but a bit more involved. In the case of time-to-event data, there are a large number of papers summarizing the relationship between hazard ratios of overall survival (OS) and progression-free survival (PFS) through meta-regression as described in the previous section. But when you have access to the patient-level data at the individual trials, then a two-stage approach is used for a more accurate estimation of the strength of the relationship between the two endpoints at both levels.

Burzowski et al. [15] developed a two-stage approach for failure time endpoints analysis that is widely used in statistical medicine literature. The R package 'surrosurv' [16] implements the R code for the two-stage approach.

16.1 Two-Stage Model for Time to Failure Endpoints

The package describes the statistical model behind the two stage-approach in its paper and implements the model in R code. Let T_{ij} be the true and S_{ij} be the surrogate endpoints for patient j in trial i. The copula function is used to model the joint probability density of both endpoints.

Burzowski et al. [15] broke down the process into steps:

- First step: Individual level

  - $h_{S_{ij}}\left(s : Z_{ij}\right) = h_{S_i}\left(s\right)e^{\alpha_j Z_{ij}}$ – exponential hazard function for

    surrogate endpoint

- $h_{T_{ij}}\left(t:Z_{ij}\right)=h_{T_i}\left(t\right)e^{\beta_j Z_{ij}}$ – exponential hazard function for
  true endpoint
- $C_\theta\left(S_{S_{ij}}\left(s\right),S_{T_{ij}}\left(t\right)\right)$ – copula function

Thus, α_i and β_i are treatment effects and Z_{ij} is the treatment indicator. The dependence function θ is re-parameterized into Kendals τ in the surrosurv package using R function tau().

The package implements three types of dependence via three copula functions: Clayton, Packet, and Hougaard. Of these the most popular is the *Clayton copula* function, which takes the following form of dependence

$$C_{\theta(u.v)=\left(u^{-\theta}+v^{-\theta}-1\right)^{-\frac{1}{\theta}}}$$

With $\theta > 0$ and Kendall's $\tau = \frac{\theta}{\theta+2}$. More details about the Clayton and other copula functions are available in the package by typing:

> vignette('copula',package='surrosurv')

- Second step: Trial level

  Mixed models are used for the estimates of treatment effects obtained from the first step as follows:

- $$\begin{pmatrix}\widehat{\alpha_i}\\\widehat{\beta_i}\end{pmatrix}=\begin{pmatrix}\alpha_i\\\beta_i\end{pmatrix}+\begin{pmatrix}\epsilon_{ai}\\\epsilon_{bi}\end{pmatrix}$$

- $$\begin{pmatrix}\widehat{\alpha_i}\\\widehat{\beta_i}\end{pmatrix}\sim N\left(\begin{pmatrix}\alpha\\\beta\end{pmatrix},D\right)\text{ with }D=\begin{pmatrix}d_b^2 & d_ad_b\rho_{trial}\\d_ad_b\rho_{trial} & d_b^2\end{pmatrix}$$

- $$\begin{pmatrix}\epsilon_{ai}\\\epsilon_{bi}\end{pmatrix}\sim N\left(\begin{pmatrix}0\\0\end{pmatrix},\Omega_i\right)\text{ with }\Omega_i=\begin{pmatrix}\omega_{ai}^2 & \omega_{ai}\omega_{bi}\rho_{\epsilon i}\\\omega_{ai}\omega_{bi}\rho_{\epsilon i} & \omega_{bi}^2\end{pmatrix}$$

where (α_i, β_i) are the true treatment effects and $(\epsilon_{ai}, \epsilon_{bi})$ are the estimation errors. Once we obtain the appropriate hazard ratio estimates from step 1 using the Clayton copula function, we can then measure the trial-level surrogacy by R_{trial}^2. Here, we have two flavors: unadjusted and adjusted. The unadjusted measure provided in the package is simply the ρ_{trial}^2, which is the squared correlation between the treatment effects (hazard ratios) of the two endpoints. We recommend using the adjusted measure, R_{trial}^2, which can be obtained using the meta-regression framework discussion earlier with weights equal to the sample size of each trial.

16.2 Example of R Code for Analyzing Gastric Cancer Data

We will analyze the 'gastadv' data set in the 'surrosurv' R package. The gastadv data set contains individual data (OR and PFS) of 4069 patients with advanced/ recurrent gastric cancer from 20 randomized trials of chemotherapy.

First, download the package from the archives directory in CRAN (compressive R archive network) website in your local directory, install the package and all its dependencies.

16.2.1 Fit Copula Model

The data set 'gastadv' in surrosurv R package will be used to fit the bivariate Copula Model and return adjusted and unadjusted log-hazard ratio estimates for OS and PFS. The data set has individual patient-level data from an advanced GATRIC meta-analysis.

```
> library(surrosurv)
> data(gastadv)
> n=table(gastadv$trialref)
> allSurroRes=surrosurv(gastadv,model='Clayton')
- Estimating model: Clayton (6.5 mins)
> predict(allSurroRes)->P #get the HR(OS) and HR(PFS)
> names(P)
[1] "Clayton.unadj" "Clayton.adj"
> P$Clayton.unadj[,1]->lHR.PFS
> P$Clayton.unadj[,2]->lHR.OS
> P$Clayton.unadj # un-adjusted log-hazard ratios for OS
and PFS.
```

By the way, here are the log hazard ratios (unadjusted):

```
> P$Clayton.unadj
   trtS     trtT
1 -0.6848 -0.227372
2 -0.4508 -0.070327
3 -0.2369 -0.208231
4 -0.2803 -0.024386
5 -0.1959 -0.225813
6 -0.5816 -0.293055
7  0.1006  0.253820
8 -0.0719 -0.185576
```

```
 9   0.1441 0.057227
10  -0.2573 -0.473316
11  -0.7444 -0.356973
12  -0.2376 -0.000661
13  -0.2008 -0.082215
14  -0.6584 -0.612046
15  -0.2503 -0.255163
16  -0.0870 0.126085
17  -0.1821 -0.238508
18  -0.2457 -0.166861
19  -0.4934 -0.180817
20  -0.4440 -0.387117
```

The 'allSurroRes' object contains the information we need to show the association between OS and PFS.

- $> R_{trial}^2$

  When we calculate the squared correlation of the hazard ratio vectors (lHR.PFS and lHR.OS) above, using the unadjusted estimates, we will match the result returned by the 'allSurroRes' object as the unadjusted R_{trial}^2.

  If we had extracted the adjusted estimates of hazard ratios instead and computed ρ^2, we would match the adjusted estimate of R_{trial}^2 in the object.

- R_{indiv}^2

For the individual-level measure of association, we will consider the estimates of Kendall's Tau in the 'allSurroRes' object. Kendall's Tau ϵ (0, 1) and the value of 0.61 using the bivariate Clayton copula denotes moderate strength of association.

Here is the printout of the object to check your answers against:

```
> allSurroRes
                kTau  R2
Clayton unadj   0.61  0.45
Clayton adj     0.61  0.41
```

16.2.2 Fit Weighted Least Squares Model

We fit weighted least squares model on Adjusted estimates of the log hazard ratios for PFS and OS.

The adjusted log-hazard ratios for OS and PFS from R object P$Clayton.adj will be used to fit Weighted Least Square (WLS) model with weight to be the sample size for each trial (total 20 trials).

```
> P$Clayton.adj[,1]->lHR.PFS
> P$Clayton.adj[,2]->lHR.OS
> M=lm(lHR.OS~lHR.PFS, weights=n)
> summary(M)
```

Coefficients:

Estimate Std. Error t value Pr(>|t|)

(Intercept) -0.03887 0.03660 -1.062 0.30223

lPFS 0.47948 0.12956 3.701 0.00164**

Signif. codes: 0 '***' 0.001 '**' 0.01 '*' 0.05 '.' 0.1 ' ' 1

Residual standard error: 1.197 on 18 degrees of freedom

Multiple R-squared: 0.4321, Adjusted R-squared: 0.4006

F-statistic: 13.7 on 1 and 18 degrees of freedom, *P* value: 0.001636

We see that the measure of association is 0.43, and once again points to a low-moderate degree of associations

Extract MSPE (mean squared error of the predictions):

```
> M=lm(lHR.OS~lHR.PFS, weights=n)
> library(DAAG)
> RISK=data.frame(n, lHR=lHR.OS, lPFSHR=lHR.PFS)
> colnames(RISK) = c("Num. Trial","n", "lHR", "lPFSHR")
> cv = CVlm(data=RISK, form.lm=formula(lHR~lPFSHR,
weight s=n),m=nrow(RISK),seed=617, plotit = FALSE)
> MSPE = attr(cv, "ms")
. . . . . .
```

```
> MSPE
[1] 0.0271
```

Extract MSE (mean squared error):

```
> library(ISLR); library(modelr);library(purrr)
> loocv.data=crossv_kfold(RISK, k=nrow(RISK))
> loocv.models=map(loocv.data$train,~lm(1HR~1PFSHR,
weights=n, data=RISK))
> loocv.mse=map2_dbl(loocv.models, loocv.data$test, mse)
> MSE=mean(loocv.mse)
```

> MSE

[1] 0.0223

16.2.3 WLS Regression Plot

The following plot was from the WLS regression of OS log HR on PFS log HR across all trials with the sample sizes of the trails as the weights (Figure 16.1).

```
> WLS_stats = data.frame(R_squared = round(summary(M)$r.
squared,2),
+           MSPE = round(attr(cv, "ms"),2),
+           MSE = round(MSE,2))
> plot(x=RISK$1PFSHR, y=RISK$1HR, xlim=c(-1,1),
ylim=c(-1,1), type="n",
+    main="WLS regression across all trials\n gastadv
     data, surrosurv package",
+ xlab="PFS log HR", ylab = "OS log HR")
> points(x=RISK$1PFSHR, y=RISK$1HR, cex=n/min(n, na.rm=T),
  col="blue")
> abline(M$coefficients, lwd=1.8)
> legend("top", paste("WLS R Square = ", round(summary(M)
$r.squared,2)), bty="n")
```

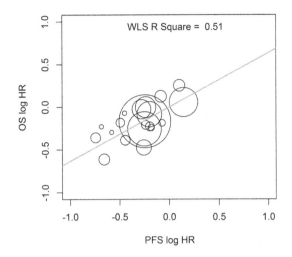

FIGURE 16.1
WLS regression across all trials gastadv data, surrosurv package.

17

Examining the Proportion of Treatment Effect in AIDS Clinical Trials

Many investigators have contributed statistical methodology toward validating change in CD4 cell count as a surrogate endpoint for clinical outcome in HIV-infected patients. I will focus on one paper in particular that made a significant contribution in this disease area for this surrogate endpoint. Hughes et al. [10] outline two methods for showing surrogacy in their seminal paper as: (a) approach 1: this is the within-trial statistical approach of calculating proportion of treatment effect (PTE) explained by the surrogate and (b) approach 2: across-trial approach: this is the statistical approach of meta-analysis of pooling information from several trials.

17.1 Definition

First, let us define the PTE as a tool to measure the level of surrogacy between S (surrogate endpoint) and T (true endpoint).

If we fit two models where Z_j is the treatment indicator for the jth patient:

- $T_j = \mu_T + \beta Z_j + \epsilon_{T_j}$
- $T_j = \mu + \beta_S Z_j + \gamma S_j + \varepsilon$

then PTE $\equiv \frac{\hat{\beta} - \hat{\beta}_S}{\hat{\beta}}$ which is the proportion of the treatment effect on the true endpoint explained by the surrogate endpoint. Note this framework of two models can be used for any number of outcomes (continuous, ordinal, binary, time to event) and predictors.

If PTE is 0, when $\hat{\beta} - \hat{\beta}_S = 0$, or two coefficients are equal, the surrogate endpoint plays no role in explaining the treatment effect on the true endpoint. Conversely, if PTE is 1, when $\hat{\beta}_S = 0$, then the surrogate endpoint absorbs the entire treatment effect on the true endpoint. It is clear from the definition above, however, that PTE is not constrained between 0 and 1. The quantity can be negative or even larger than 1. There are several papers that introduce other parameters that have better properties; however, PTE is one of the most ubiquitous parameters used to show surrogacy.

17.2 Background of the Two Approaches

Hughes et al. [10] evaluated initial changes in CD4 cell count as a surrogate endpoint for clinical outcome in HIV-infected patients. The true endpoint, T, was progression to AIDS or death (or death alone) after 6 months that was explained by the surrogate endpoint, S, which is the change in CD4 cell count during the first 6 months.

The PTE and its corresponding 95% confidence interval (CI) were plotted in Figure 1.a and 1.b of their paper.

The 95% confidence interval formula for this setting – involving time-to-event clinical outcome data – has been derived by the methodology developed by Lin et al. [17] and specified in formula (5) of their paper.

17.3 Approach 1

Following this methodology, Hughes et al. [10] fit two Cox proportional hazards models to the data from AIDS clinical trials:

- Model 1

$$l\left(t|\,Z\right) = l_1\left(t\right)e^{\beta Z + \gamma W(t)}$$

  where this is a model with the surrogate endpoint (e.g., CD4 count in AIDS/HIV trial) and $W(t)$ is the potential surrogate covariate (t denotes that the surrogate endpoint could be time varying).

- Model 2

$$l\left(t|\,Z\right) = l_2\left(t\right)e^{\alpha Z}$$

  where this is a model without the surrogate endpoint.

Note $\alpha, \beta,$ and γ are the unknown regression parameters. Lin et al. provide derivations for setting a system of equations (of the partial likelihood score function) to 0 and obtaining the solutions as the estimates of these parameters.

Our parameter of interest to measure surrogacy, the PTE, is defined by

$$\hat{p} = 1 - \frac{\hat{\beta}}{\hat{\alpha}}$$

The authors use the delta method to show that the random variable

$$\sqrt{n}\left(\hat{p}-p^*\right) \sim Normal\left(0,\sigma^2\right)$$

where $\sigma^2 = \frac{V_\beta}{\alpha^{*2}} + \frac{\left(\beta^*\right)^2 V_\alpha}{\alpha^{*4}} - 2\frac{\left(\beta^*\right)V_{\alpha\beta}}{\alpha^{*3}}$ and V_α, V_β, and $V_{\alpha\beta}$ are the variances and covariances of $\sqrt{n}\hat{\alpha}$ and $\sqrt{n}\hat{\beta}$.

Beth Zamboni in her PhD dissertation [16] explained how Wei et al. used the marginal hazard model for multiple events data to get the correct estimates for the variances and covariances. Models 1 and 2 cannot hold at the same time, but Lin et al. [17] show that $\hat{p}$ is still a useful measure of the PTE explained by the surrogate – especially when $\hat{\alpha}, \hat{\beta}$ are close to their true values. Lin et al. mention a nifty trick whereby they create artificial bivariate data to represent models 1 and 2 – doubling the data set in dimension and fitting the regular cox proportional hazards model to obtain the correlation between the parameters. Zamboni in her dissertation shows us how to do it.

Zamboni elucidated the algorithm by Lin et al. [17] of artificially constructing bivariate survival data as following:

1. Construct double sets of the survival data, including the dependent variable and covariate data.

   a. First set will contain the complete survival data; and treatment as the first covariate (α coefficient); dummy variable 0 as the second covariate; and dummy variable 0 as the third covariate.

   b. Second set will contain the complete survival data; and dummy variable 0 as the first covariate; treatment as the second covariate (β coefficient); and surrogate marker as the third covariate (γ coefficient).

2. Use regular function coxph() from R to analyze the data and obtain estimates for α, β, V_α, V_β, and $V_{\alpha\beta}$.

3. Use the strata option to distinguish the two sets and use subject ID as a cluster.

4. Using standard asymptotic normal theory, construct confidence interval for p as

$$\hat{p} \pm z_{1-\varphi/2}\sqrt{\frac{\hat{\sigma}^2}{n}}.$$

17.3.1 R Code for Approach #1

I provide the R code below to do the computations:

```
>library(sqldf)
>library(survival)
```

#The 'aids' data set is available in R package 'mdhglm'. You can use any data set that has the survival data and the surrogate biomarker.

```
>head(aids)
patient Time death  CD4 obstime drug gender prevOI  AZT   start stop event
1   1 16.97  0 10.677078   0  ddC  male  AIDS intolerance  0 6.0 0
2   2 19.00  0  6.324555   0  ddI  male noAIDS intolerance 0 6.0 0
3   3 18.53  1  3.464102   0  ddI  female AIDS intolerance 0 2.0 0
4   4 12.70  0  3.872983   0  ddC  male   AIDS failure     0 2.0 0
5   5 15.13  0  7.280110   0  ddI  male   AIDS failure     0 2.0 0
6   6  1.90  1  4.582576   0  ddC  female AIDS failure     0 1.9 1
```

#Now create the two data sets for Model 1 and Model 2

```
aids1=data.frame(aids[,c(1,2,3)],x1=ifelse(aids$drug=='ddC',
1,0),
     x2=rep(0,nrow(aids)),w=rep(0,nrow(aids)),etype=rep(1,nrow
     (aids)))
>aids2=data.frame(aids[,c(1,2,3)],x1=rep(0,nrow(aids)),
     x2=ifelse(aids$drug=='ddC',1,0),w=aids$CD4,etype=rep(2,
     nrow(aids)))
>aids1[,1]=as.numeric(as.character(aids1[,1]))
>head(aids1)
patient Time death x1 x2 w etype
1       1 16.97    0  1  0 0    1
2       2 19.00    0  0  0 0    1
3       3 18.53    1  0  0 0    1
4       4 12.70    0  1  0 0    1
5       5 15.13    0  0  0 0    1
6       6  1.90    1  1  0 0    1


>aids2[,1]=as.numeric(as.character(aids2[,1]))
>head(aids2)
patient  Time death x1 x2       w etype
1        1 16.97    0  0  1 10.677078    2
2        2 19.00    0  0  0  6.324555    2
3        3 18.53    1  0  0  3.464102    2
4        4 12.70    0  0  1  3.872983    2
5        5 15.13    0  0  0  7.280110    2
6        6  1.90    1  0  1  4.582576    2
```

```
#Stack aids1 and aids2 together
>aids3=sqldf("select * from aids1 union select * from aids2")
>aids3[,1]=as.factor(as.character(aids3[,1]))
>head(aids3)
patient  Time death x1 x2       w etype
1          1 16.97    0  0  1 10.677078    2
2          1 16.97    0  1  0  0.000000    1
3          2 19.00    0  0  0  0.000000    1
4          2 19.00    0  0  0  6.324555    2
5          3 18.53    1  0  0  0.000000    1
6          3 18.53    1  0  0  3.464102    2

>fitCOX=coxph(Surv(Time,death)~(x1+x2+w)*strata(etype)+
cluster(patient),data=aids3)
>summary(fitCOX)
>alpha=fitCOX$coef[1]
>beta=fitCOX$coef[2]

>V.alpha=fitCOX$var[1]
>V.beta=fitCOX$var[8]
>V.alpha.beta=fitCOX$var[7]

>p=1-(beta/alpha)
>sigma.sq=((V.beta/alpha^2)+(((beta^2)*V.alpha)/alpha^4)
-(2*beta*V.alpha.beta/alpha^3))
>sigma=sqrt(sigma.sq)

>lower.ci=p-1.96*sigma
>upper.ci=p+1.96*sigma
```

The Hughes investigation plotted the estimated PTE($\hat{p}$) and corresponding 95% interval of each trial in a forest plot (Figure 1.a and 1.b). Some of the estimates were outside the range of (0,1). Two reasons were given, first the poor precision of the confidence interval of PTE; second PTE itself can be signaling that treatment can have a deleterious effect on disease progression through a mechanism of action not captured by the surrogate. However, majority of the estimated PTE's were above 0. In addition to producing the within-trial PTE estimates and CI's for each trial, Hughes et al. then produced a weighted average of the PTE with weights equal to the inverse of the square of its standard error. The reason the inverse is chosen as the precision of the estimate of each proportion (PTE) is that more variability will lead to less weight being given to that proportion. The weighted average for the PTE in the Hughes paper was small (0.16; 95% CI, 0.07–0.26), which suggested a modest proportion explained by the surrogate. Remember that the disease outcome is time to progression to AIDS or death after six months of treatment; and the surrogate is change in CD4 cell count during the first 6 months. Perhaps, considering CD4 cell count as a time-varying covariate would increase the strength of the surrogacy (magnitude of PTE). Nevertheless, the evidence already points to a modest degree of surrogacy for 6 months of change in CD4 cell count.

In general, one may consider the lower bound of the confidence interval of the PTE to be above 0 to find relevance in the surrogate and perhaps close to 0.5 to be a strong surrogate. The strength considered relevant is subject to the disease area and to the disease-treatment research stage, with later stages requiring more evidence of strength.

One last point to consider when comparing the individual-study level PTE estimates, 95%CI's as well as computing the weighted average PTE, is to remember to order the treatments in the trial in a similar manner. For example, the lowest level of the treatment variable assigned to placebo or control group and so on. This point is also important in computing the study-level statistics summarizing treatment effect on surrogate endpoints and clinical outcomes – and will be used in the following approach.

17.4 Approach 2

This is largely a meta-analytic framework across trials for investigating pairwise association between treatment effect on disease outcome as well as on the surrogate endpoint. In our example, the log hazard ratio for progression to AIDS or death comparing test and control treatments was one of the disease outcomes (γ_i); the difference by treatment group in mean change of CD4 cell counts from baseline to 6 months (x_i) and their standard errors (s_i) were the surrogate endpoint measures.

17.4.1 Linear Regression

We can first think of the analysis as a simple ordinary least squares (OLS) regression:

$$\gamma_i = \alpha + \beta x_i + \varepsilon_i$$

where ε_i measures the variations of the true log hazard ratios for the ith trial from that predicted by the true difference in mean change in CD4 cell count by treatment.

In order for the surrogacy to be relevant, we expect $\beta \neq 0$ with statistical significance. In addition, since no difference in mean CD4 cell counts should reflect no change in log hazard ratios, we expect $\alpha \approx 0$ (both are specified in the Prentice criterion [6]). If, however, this second condition does not quite hold, it means that the surrogate does not explain all of the treatment effect on the disease outcome and some alternative mechanism to the clinical outcome, is also mediating the treatment effect. Thus, the results of the analysis should be carefully interpreted.

We can fit this linear regression above with the weights as the inverse of the standard errors (s_i) of the surrogate measures of the ith comparison. In this example, each comparison is a trial where the outcome variable and the predictor variable could be computed or is available from each trial. If a trial did not collect the data to compute the chosen outcome and predictor (surrogate) variable (e.g., subject's 6 months change in CD4 cell count), then that trial needs to be excluded from the meta-analysis. One can easily see, therefore, that a sufficient number of trials needs to have been run for this analysis to be valid.

Note there is another problem with running an ordinary or weighted linear regression on the trial level data. The predictor variable is not known for each trial but is rather estimated. Thus, a Bayesian approach could be taken to correctly model the metadata properly accounting for the variability of the estimates.

17.4.2 Bayesian Linear Regression

Before we introduce Bayesian linear regression here, first let us refer to the methodology introduced by Daniels and Hughes [19] and used by in this analysis approach we have been discussing. The authors introduce a new parameter, τ^2, which measures the variability of the departure terms ε_i. Thus, all three parameters are important to estimate in evaluating a surrogate endpoint. When $\beta \neq 0$ we will need to model τ^2, which will give us an estimate of the heterogeneity of the treatment effects from the different trials. A vague prior distribution is used on α and β and a shrinkage prior distribution for τ^2 is specified in the methodology proposed by Daniels and Hughes [19]. The 95% prediction intervals were computed for all three parameters. The authors used Markov chain Monte Carlo (MCMC) techniques, specifically the Gibbs sample, for the computations and the details are further described in that paper.

Hughes et al. [15] computed the prediction intervals using this methodology mentioned above to show that when treatment group differences in the mean change of CD4 cell count at 6 months is zero and its standard error is zero, the predicted hazard ratio is approximately 1. Higher treatment group differences in the mean change of CD4 cell count at 6 months with a higher standard error (imprecision in estimates) to show survival benefit. This is expected and is shown very nicely in the numerical results presented in Table 2 of the paper [11].

Now let us discuss the implementation of Bayesian linear regression using the R package 'bayesreg'. There are many packages in R that would enable the reader to conduct Bayesian linear regression. However, I choose this package for the relative ease of use. The 'bayesreg' package features Bayesian linear regression with Gaussian or heavy-tailed error models and Bayesian logistic regression with ridge, lasso, and other regularization estimators. Makalic and Schmidt [20] introduce the hierarchical framework in their paper through seven key equations consisting of two key groups: (i) the model for the

sampling distribution of the data (1)–(3) and (ii) the prior distributions for
the regression coefficients (5)–(7). The details are in their paper where they
construct statistical models for both the data and the prior distributions from
exchangeable Gaussian variance mixture distributions.

The R package 'metamisc' contains the trial-level summaries for the 15 trials included in the analysis in Daniels and Hughes [19] methodology for
evaluating surrogacy for CD4 cell count at 6 months.

The Daniels data comprises 15 phase II/III randomized clinical trials of the
HIV Disease Section of the Adult AIDS Clinical Trials Group of the National
Institutes of Health, which had data available as of May 1996, which had at
least 6 months follow-up on some patients and in which at least one patient
developed AIDS or died. The data were previously used by Daniels and Hughes
(1997) to assess whether the change in CD4 cell count is a surrogate for time to
either development of AIDS or death in drug trials of patients with HIV.

17.4.2.1 R Code

The R code is given below:

```
>library(bayesreg)
>library(metamisc)
>logHR=Daniels$Y1 #Read in the Daniels and Hughes paper - AIDS
- CD4 data set of 15 trials
>DD_ChgCD4=Daniels$Y2 #Treatment differences for the log
hazard ratio
          #for the development of AIDS or death over 2 years
>o=order(DD_ChgCD4) #Difference in mean change in CD4 cell count
        #between baseline and 6 month for studies of the AIDS
          Clinical Trial Group
>logHR=logHR[o]
>DD_ChgCD4=DD_ChgCD4[o]
>df = data.frame(DD_ChgCD4,logHR)
# Gaussian ridge
>rv.G <- bayesreg(logHR~., df, model = "gaussian",
prior = "ridge", n.samples = 1e3)
# Student-t ridge
>rv.t <- bayesreg(logHR~., df, model = "t", prior =
"ridge", t.dof = 5, n.samples = 1e3)
# Plot the different estimates with credible intervals
>plot(df$DD_ChgCD4, df$logHR, xlab="Diff in Mean Change in
CD4 @6 months",   ylim=range(logHR),ylab="log HR")
>yhat_G <- predict(rv.G, df, bayes.avg=TRUE)
>lines(df$DD_ChgCD4, yhat_G[,1], col="blue", lwd=2.5)
>lines(df$DD_ChgCD4, yhat_G[,3], col="blue", lwd=1,
lty="dashed")
>lines(df$DD_ChgCD4, yhat_G[,4], col="blue", lwd=1,
lty="dashed")
>yhat_t <- predict(rv.t, df, bayes.avg=TRUE)
```

```
>lines(df$DD_ChgCD4, yhat_t[,1], col="darkred", lwd=2.5)
>lines(df$DD_ChgCD4, yhat_t[,3], col="darkred",
lwd=1, lty="dashed")
>lines(df$DD_ChgCD4, yhat_t[,4], col="darkred",
lwd=1, lty="dashed")
>legend(0,-1,c("Gaussian","Student-t (dof=5)"),lty=c(1,1),
col=c("blue","darkred"),
lwd=c(2.5,2.5), cex=0.7)
>summary(rv.G)
```

The plot produced by the above code shows the different estimates and their prediction intervals (Figure 17.1).

The summary of the Bayesian linear regression shows that (i) even though the estimated slope is close to 0, its 95% credible interval for the slope estimate excludes 0; but that of the intercept estimate includes 0. See the table below.

Bayesreg: Bayesian Penalized Regression Estimation ver. 1.1 (c) Daniel F Schmidt, Enes Makalic. 2016-9								
Bayesian Gaussian ridge regression			Number of obs = 15					
			Number of vars = 1					
MCMC Samples = 1000			std(Error) = 0.35275					
MCMC Burnin = 1000			R-squared = 0.6042					
MCMC Thinning = 5			WAIC = 6.2506					
Parameter		mean(Coef)	std(Coef)	[95% Cred. Interval]		tStat	Rank	ESS
DD_ChgCD4		−0.01364	0.00454	−0.02221	−0.00276	−3.006	1 **	83.8
_cons		0.06192	0.12686	−0.24174	0.30364	.	.	.

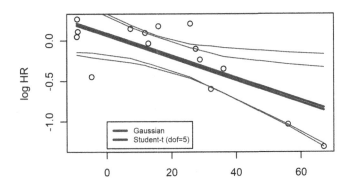

FIGURE 17.1
Bayes Linear Regression Difference in mean change in CD4 (x) vs log hazard ratio (y).

18

Concluding Remarks

The section on surrogate endpoint gives several examples of how to evaluate a variable as a surrogacy measure of a clinical endpoint. Most sections are accompanied by R code for analysis. It takes time, effort, collaboration, and investment to establish a surrogate variable in a particular disease area. Examples in oncology and HIV/AIDS are given to illustrate how data were pooled across trials to establish the surrogate. The analyses are useful even when a regulatory decision on surrogate endpoint is not imminent. While pharmacodynamic markers are used to measure target engagement for the drug and clinical outcomes are used to measure treatment efficacy for the disease, many biomarkers will have their utility fall anywhere in between. For example, if a drug is to move forward from Phase II to Phase III, a biomarker which serves like a preliminary surrogate marker is useful in making an informed decision for the drug manufacturer about the magnitude of clinical benefit expected from clinical endpoint.

References

1. https://en.wikipedia.org/wiki/Surrogate_endpoint
2. https://www.cancer.gov/publications/dictionaries/cancer-terms/def/surrogate-endpoint
3. https://www.bcrf.org/blog/asco-2017-clinical-trial-updates-early-stage-breast-cancer
3a. https://www.fda.gov/Drugs/DevelopmentApprovalProcess/DevelopmentResources/ucm606684.htm
3b. https://www.fda.gov/Drugs/DevelopmentApprovalProcess/DevelopmentResources/ucm613636.htm
3c. https://www.fda.gov/Drugs/DevelopmentApprovalProcess/DevelopmentResources/ucm613636.htm
4. https://www.focr.org/clinical-trial-endpoints
5. https://www.publichealth.pitt.edu/Portals/0/BIOSTAT/Abberbock_etd_August2017.pdf?ver=2017-10-23-081615-487
6. Prentice RL. (1989). Surrogate endpoints in clinical trials: Definition and operational criteria. *Stat. Med.*, 8(4):431–440.
6a. Freedman LS, Graubard BI, Schatzkin A. (1992). Statistical validation of intermediate endpoints for chronic diseases. *Stat. Med.*, 11(2):167–178.

6b. Alonso A, Molenberghs G. (2007). Surrogate marker evaluation from an information theory perspective. *Biometrics*, 63:180–186.

6c. Buyse M, Molenberghs G, Burzykowski T, Renard D, Geys H. (2000). The validation of surrogate endpoints in meta-analyses of randomized experiments. *Biostatistics*, 1(1):49–67.

6d. Burzykowski T, Molenberghs G, Buyse M. (2006). *The Evaluation of Surrogate Endpoints*. Springer Science & Business Media https://www.springer.com/gp/book/9780387202778.

7. Sherrill B, Kaye JA, Sandin R, Cappelleri JC, Chen C. (2012). Review of meta-analyses evaluating surrogate endpoints for overall survival in oncology. *Onco Targets Ther.*, 5:287–296. doi:10.2147/OTT.S36683.

8. Buyse M. (2009). Use of meta-analysis for the validation of surrogate endpoints and biomarkers in cancer trials. *Cancer J.*, 15:421–425.

9. Buyse M. (2009). Contributions of meta-analyses based on individual patient data to therapeutic progress in colorectal cancer. *Int. J. Clin. Oncol.*, 14:95–101.

10. Hughes MD. (2008). Practical issues arising in an exploratory analysis evaluating progression-free survival as a surrogate endpoint for overall survival in advanced colorectal cancer. *Stat. Methods Med. Res.*, 17:487–495.

11. Burzykowski T, Buyse M. (2006). Surrogate threshold effect: An alternative measure for meta-analytic surrogate endpoint validation. *Pharm. Stat.*, 5:173–186.

12. Sargent DJ, Hayes DF. (2008). Assessing the measure of a new drug: Is survival the only thing that matters? *J. Clin. Oncol.* 26:1922–1923.

13. Wang X, Wang X, Hodgson L et al. (2017). Validation of progression-free survival as a surrogate endpoint for overall survival in malignant mesothelioma: Analysis of cancer and leukemia group B and north central cancer treatment group (Alliance) trials. *Oncologist*, 22(2):189–198.

14. Sherrill B, Kaye JA, Sandin R, Cappelleri JC, Chen C. (2012). Review of meta-analyses evaluating surrogate endpoints for overall survival in oncology. *Onco Targets Ther.*, 5:287–296.

15. Burzykowski T, Molenberghs G, Buyse M, Geys H, Renard D. (2001). Validation of surrogate end points in multiple randomized clinical trials with failure time end points. *J. R. Stat. Soc. Ser. C (Applied Statistics)*, 50(4):405–422. doi:10.1111/1467-9876.00244.

16. R package: Surrosurv: Evaluation of Failure Time Surrogate Endpoints in Individual Patient Data Meta-Analyses, Federico Rotolo, 2017, R package version 1.1.24}. https://CRAN.R-project.org/package=surrosurv

17. Lin DY, Fleming TR, de Gruttola V. (1997). Estimating the proportion of treatment effect explained by a surrogate marker. *Stat. Med.*, 16(13):1515–1527.

18. Beth Zamboni. (2015). TWISTed Survival: Identifying Surrogate Endpoints for Mortality Using QTWIST and conditional Disease Free Survival. Doctoral dissertation. University of Pittsburgh. https://pdfs.semanticscholar.org/737b/f97d5efb079c97a2b6a8e7f96d020f544fa3.pdf.

19. Daniels MJ, Hughes MD. (1997). Meta-analysis for the evaluation of potential surrogate markers. *Stat. Med.*, 16:1965–1982.

20. Makalic E, Schmidt DF. (2016). High-dimensional Bayesian regularised regression with the bayesReg package. arXiv:1611.06649 [stat. CO].

21. Fleming TR, DeMets DL. (1996). Surrogate end points in clinical trials: Are we being misled? *Ann. Intern. Med.*, 125:605–613.

Section IV

Combining Multiple Biomarkers

19

Introduction

Machine learning: field of study that gives computers the ability to learn without being explicitly programmed.

Arthur Samuel (1959)

Machine learning (ML) is the blend of computer science and statistics with the goal of learning from the data and predicting on unseen data. When multiple biomarkers are present in a data set, all being less or more important, it is possible to use ML methods to combine the biomarkers to produce a robust and sensitive signature, which predicts the clinical outcome or the treatment effect. ML is one of the most rapidly growing areas in computational sciences. In a **supervised learning** model, the algorithm learns on a data set that has the outcome variable (e.g., responder vs nonresponder or change in HbA1c levels at time t) and predicts the outcome on an unseen data set. The algorithm is judged by the accuracy of its predictions on the unseen (test) data set. An **unsupervised** model, in contrast, uses no outcome variable to train, so the algorithm learns by extracting features and patterns on its own.

The algorithm is **trained** on a data set, and judged on its prediction accuracy on a **test** data set. Thus, data sets with biomarkers, treatment, and efficacy (outcome) variable are valuable as a starting point in machine leaning. We often start with a supervised regression model to learn on the training set. This part of the book focuses on elementary ML methods with the goal of exploring multiple biomarkers. It does not provide an exhaustive list of models for exploring multiple biomarkers, but simply gives the reader an introduction to a set of commonly used ML methods they can use.

In supervised linear regression, we are interested in learning which variables (biomarkers) are important predictors of treatment effect. I do not cover the older variable selection methods in the statistical literature, for example, greedy algorithms like forward or backward stepwise selection, in the book. I encourage the readers to familiarize themselves with these traditional variable selection methods. I start with the *best subset selection* method and then introduce *regularized regression models*. Regularized Models are sometimes referred to as *Penalized Models*. This type of models adds a penalty term to the loss function we minimize when fitting the regression model. While I use the phrase 'variable selection' in the text often, it is often referred as *feature selection* in ML literature.

Not only do we want to select the important biomarkers but also build a model to discriminate between responder and nonresponder, or generate a numeric score as the clinical outcome (e.g., risk score) from the patient's observed features. Baseline features could be demographic or clinical factors, biomarker values, or changes from baseline at time t (observed prior to clinical outcome data). In order to build such a model, the useful tool of *cross-validation* is introduced. Through cross-validation, the values for the penalty term used in shrinkage-based methods (like lasso and elastic net) are chosen. The cases of linear and logistic regression modeling for variable selection and prediction are discussed in the following chapters. The Cox regression model has been enabled with regularization procedures through the R package 'coxnet', but I do not discuss them below. For a general introduction on elementary ML methods, I recommend the classic text by Hastie et al. [4].

The role of modeling interactions is important in pharmaceutical statistics. In this case, we are interested in treatment–biomarker interactions. I describe a regularized regression method for learning interaction effects.

Classification and regression trees (CART) procedures are described as tools for building interpretable interactions between variables for explaining the outcome in biomarker data sets. Cluster analysis methods are included when we are employing unsupervised learning on data sets without labels (outcome variable). Recently, graphical models have been gaining interest in modeling biomedical data. These models could reveal important variables and their interrelationships in multivariate biomarker data sets.

All the methods introduced in this chapter are applicable in scenarios where the curse of dimensionality is present (p>>n). While clinical trials collect many biomarkers, we often find ourselves in this scenario where the sample size is small.

Again, this part of the book contains a sample of the commonly used ML techniques for looking at multiple biomarkers in clinical trials. Reading the examples will give the user a starting point into the vast universe of ML tools that can be employed in analyzing biomarkers in the era of big data.

20

Regression-Based Models

20.1 Best Subset Selection

Multiple biomarkers are often available in the clinical trial data set, where we might perform the exercise of

1. Identifying which biomarkers are associated with the disease outcome and build a parsimonious, multivariate model for predicting the dependent variable
2. Combining the biomarkers into a single model to predict the dependent variable (e.g., disease outcome)
3. Estimating prediction error using the model's predictions in an independent validation data set
4. Interpreting the association of the biomarkers to the dependent variable (e.g., disease outcome), or the disease-modifying nature of the drug through modulation of the biomarkers

The biomarkers can be measured at baseline and hence would be predictive in nature, or you could be looking at changes from baseline at a certain timepoint t. The data set we consider here is hence cross-sectional in nature where time is fixed. The disease outcome can be continuous, binary, categorical, or survival. In a collection of biomarkers, we do want to eliminate the ones that are not associated with the outcome of interest based on statistical reasoning. To this end, historically, statisticians have used stepwise selection processes (e.g., forward, backward, or both) to identify important variables. Yet, this procedure yields in based estimates of regression coefficients (upward in magnitude), standard errors and p-values (downward in magnitude). More recent methods include subset selection in linear regression and logistic regression, via (a) various information criteria or (b) cross-validation (CV).

20.1.1 Data Set

There are 99 subjects in this synthetic data set representing a clinical data set. We are interested in identifying biomarkers, which may be predictive of a safety signal, y_i. Assume everyone is treated with the drug. There are seven features (biomarkers) and five demographic variables. Each of these variables are numeric. Fifteen subjects had the toxic response to the treatment in the trial.

20.1.2 R Analysis – Preprocessing

We begin by exploring the distribution of the biomarkers. This step is about cleaning and manipulating the data matrix as necessary.

```
library(caret)
library(ggplot2)

#if (!requireNamespace("BiocManager", quietly = TRUE))
#  install.packages("BiocManager")

#BiocManager::install("scater")
library(scater)      #for multiplot on same page

bm=read.csv("bm.csv",header=TRUE)
B=bm[,c(3:9)]

plot_data_column = function (data, column) {
    ggplot(data, aes_string(x = column)) +
    geom_histogram(fill = "darkgrey") +
    xlab(column)
    }

myplots <- lapply(colnames(B), plot_data_column, data = B)

multiplot(plotlist = myplots, layout=matrix(c(1,2,3,4,5,6,7,7),
    nrow=4, byrow=TRUE))
```

The output is provided in Figure 20.1, and we see that the biomarkers are skewed right. Therefore, we will log-transform the biomarker data for further analyses.

Since we assume that the number of comparisons will be small in the context of the number of biomarkers in a typical clinical biomarkers, relative to genomics data where there are hundreds or thousands of biomarkers, we will use FWER (family-wise error rate) to control the type I error rate of 0.05. The Holm–Bonferroni correction takes the original alpha level and divides it by the total number of comparisons subtracted by the rank of the p-value plus one. This is more powerful than Bonferroni, which is equally punitive to each comparison.

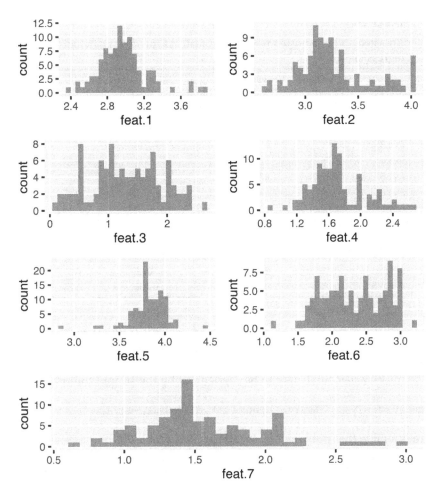

FIGURE 20.1
Histogram of features (predictors).

20.1.3 R – Univariate and Multivariate Analyses

The code for univariate analysis via R function 'glm' for logistic regression is given below. We extract the p-values and use the 'Holm' procedure for adjustment due to making multiple univariate comparisons.

```
univcoefs = lapply(bm[3:ncol(bm)],function(x)
          summary(glm(bm$y~x,family="binomial"))$coef)


pvals=NULL;
for (i in 1:ncol(bm[,-c(1:2)])){
    pvals=rbind(pvals,(univcoefs[[i]][2,4]))
    }
p.adjust(pvals,"holm")
```

TABLE 20.1

Adjusted and unadjusted p-values for features (predictors) in logistic regression

Marker	Univariate Coef	Univariate P Value	Adj p (Holm)	Multivariate Coef	Multivariate P Value
feat.1	−2.1	0.1	0.8	0.53	0.88
feat.2	−0.24	0.78	1	−0.25	0.94
feat.3	−5.9	0	0	−7.16	0
feat.4	−0.78	0.37	1	9.11	0.07
feat.5	0.39	0.79	1	−1.27	0.7
feat.6	0.04	0.94	1	1.78	0.57
feat.7	−2.09	0.02	0.22	−3.15	0.32
demo.1	0.04	0.05	0.45	0.08	0.19
demo.2	0.02	0.39	1	−0.07	0.3
demo.3	0.02	0.02	0.22	0.06	0.11
demo.4	−0.15	0.34	1	0.29	0.39
demo.5	−0.05	0.38	1	−0.06	0.74

When you exponentiate the coefficient of variable X (feature 1, e.g.), you find the factor, the odds of Y (safety event) gets multiplied by, for 1 unit increase in X.

The multivariate analysis can be carried out by the simple command:

```
summary(glm(y~.,family="binomial",data=bm[,-1]))
```

Here is a table that puts the results all together (Table 20.1).

Biomarkers (features) 3, 7, and demo 3 seem to be significant or marginally significant correlates of the odds of having a safety event in both the univariate and multivariate analysis. The coefficients are different of course, both in meaning and in value, because the univariate and multivariate models are different.

Let us now evaluate the process of variable selection.

20.1.4 Variable Selection via R Package 'bestglm'

The variable selection from exhaustively searching all combinations of covariates is called *best subset selection* in the regression setting. The R library 'bestglm' [1] provides very efficient algorithms for searching for the best subsets. The authors provide vignettes [2,3], which show several examples of this package.

The function 'bestglm' uses the simple exhaustive search algorithm [38] for glm and the regsubsets function in the leaps package to find the glm models with smallest sum of squares or deviances for size k = 0, 1, …, p, where p=# of terms in the model. Size k = 0 corresponds to intercept only. The exhaustive search requires more computer time but this is usually not an issue when p <= 10. This is an important limitation to remember for this method which explores all possible subsets which involves considering 2^p models. This exponential time algorithm is NP-hard.

Back to bestglm(), you can force a coefficient to be included as well. Let us name the options for model selection included in the package. Various information criteria are offered: AIC, BIC, extended BIC methods, like, BIC_g, BIC_q [3], and many variations of the CV procedure. I focus on CV in this book as it is a general approach when you do not know whether model is finite or infinite dimensional or the form of the relationship with the covariates is linear or additive. Let us remind the reader that both AIC and BIC assess the model fit penalized by the number of estimated parameters, but BIC penalizes more than AIC [4].

$$AIC = -2\log(L) + 2p$$

$$BIC = -2\log(L) + p\log(n)$$

where L is the value of the likelihood, n is the number of recorded measurements, and p is the number of estimated parameters.

Here, p is the number of predictors and n is the number of observations. If the goal is to produce a sparse model, then it might be better to use BIC.

Even though I will focus mainly on CV in the book, I want to first give the reader the results from using the BIC_q selection criterion offered in the package on the 'bm' data set.

20.1.4.1 The BIC$_q$ Criterion

The BIC_q criterion [3] is derived by assuming a Bernoulli prior for the parameters. Each parameter has a priori probability of q of being included, where $q \in [0, 1]$. With this prior, the resulting information criterion can be written,

$$BIC_q = D + K\log(n) - 2k\log\left(\frac{q}{1-q}\right)$$

When q = 1/2, the BICq is equivalent to the BIC, while q = 0 and q = 1 correspond to selecting the models with k = p and k = 0, respectively. For q = 0, the penalty is taken to be $-\infty$ and so no parameters are selected and similarly for q = 1, the full model with all covariates is selected. Xu and McLeod [2] derive an interval estimate for q that is based on a confidence probability α,

$0 < \alpha < 1$. This parameter may be set by the optional argument qLevel = α. The default setting is with $\alpha = 0.99$.

The R code and results are below:

```
> library(bestglm)
Loading required package: leaps
> ######Best subset selection #############
> Xy<-cbind(as.data.frame(bm[,3:ncol(bm)]), safe=bm$y)
> out <- bestglm(Xy, IC="BICq")
```

The object 'out' contains the following result:

	Estimate	Std. Err	t value	Pr(>|t|)
(Intercept)	-0.061	0.138	-0.441	0.660
feat.3	-0.499	0.054	-9.259	0.000
feat.4	0.477	0.093	5.127	0.000
demo.3	0.002	0.001	2.767	0.007

We see that the penalized algorithm chose three covariates. One issue is that if we had a large number of predictors, p, then the information criteria may give overfitted results.

20.1.4.2 Cross-Validation

CV is a data-splitting procedure, which repeatedly splits the data into a training and a test set. The goal is to identify the optimal model. Still, ideally, an independent data set is desirable to estimate the chosen model.

Leave-1-out CV is asymptotically equivalent to AIC (and Mallows' Cp) [5]. Leave-k-out CV asymptotically equivalent to BIC for well-chosen k. Increasing k tends to simpler models. Note that CV with large k requires estimation of many parameters with little data if your sample size is small. Still, CV is the preferred approach for identifying the optimal model.

One of the several variations of CV offered in the R package 'bestglm' is 'delete-d CV'. The procedure, introduced by Shao [6], takes random samples of size d to be used as the validation set, where d is set to

$$d = n\left(1 - \left(\log n - 1\right) - 1\right)$$

where n is the number of observations = 99.

Many validation sets are generated in this way and the complementary part of the data is used each time as the training set. Typically, 1000 validation sets are used. This is the value of d used in the default settings when information criterion IC = 'CV' option is used.

```
> set.seed(650)
> bestglm(Xy, IC="CV")
```

The command gives the same output for this data as the bestglm() output above.

Again, we see that the same variables have been chosen through delete-d-CV approach.

Hastie et al. [4] discuss K-fold CV. With this method, the data are divided, randomly, into K folds of approximately equal size. For the *k*th part, we fit the model to the other $K-1$ parts of the data and calculate the prediction error of the fitted model when predicting the *k*th part of the data. We do this for $k = 1, 2, ..., K$ and combine the K estimates of prediction error. Then, the CV estimate of prediction error is

$$CV(\hat{f}) = \frac{1}{n}\sum_{i=1}^{N} L\left(y_i, \hat{f}^{-k(i)}(x_i)\right),$$

where N is the number of data points, L is the loss function, (x_i, y_i) is the *i*th data point, $k(i)$ is the function that maps the observation *i* to the group *k* it belongs, and $\hat{f}^{-k(i)}$ is the model trained with the data set excluding the $k(i)$ part. In our case, the x_i is the biomarker value, y_i is the safety event occurrence indicator, the function f is the logistic function, and L is the logistic loss.

The choice of K is a statistical topic of interest.

- When K = 2, we are in the split-sample scenario. The error estimates are biased upward because only half the data is used to train the model.
- When K = n, we are in the leave-one-out-CV scenario. Here, the CV error estimates have high variance, since we are averaging many positively correlated estimates.
- Usually K = 5 or 10 is sufficient for most data sets. The CV error estimates are less correlated and the error estimates have similar variance.

We produce plots of prediction errors by subset size below as shown in the 'bestglm' package'.

McLeod and Xu [1] in the package 'bestglm' provides code to reproduce from Hastie [4], page 62, Figure 3.3. Figure 20.2 illustrates how the one-standard deviation rule is applied to model selection (K = 10):

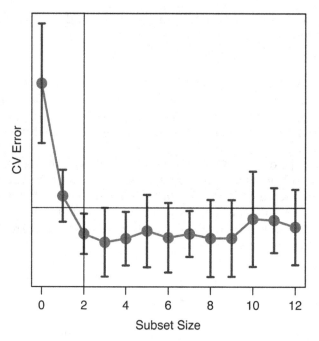

FIGURE 20.2
Cross-validation error vs subset size.

The 'one SD rule' is defined as the smallest value of prediction error yielding a CV error no more than one standard error above its minimum value. The vertical dashed line is where the minimum occurs, and the horizontal line shows the one SD rule. The one standard error rule is an alternative way of choosing θ (best subset size and variables) from the CV curve. We start with the usual estimate $\hat{\theta} = \operatorname{argmin} \theta \in \{\theta_1,...,\theta_m\}$ for $CV(\theta)$ and we move θ in the direction of increasing regularization until it ceases to be true that $CV(\theta) \leq CV(\hat{\theta}) + SE(\hat{\theta})$. Thus, we take the simplest (most regularized) model whose error is within one standard error of the minimal error.

Specifically, for two-class classification, where each $y_i \in \{0, 1\}$, and we use the 0-1 loss function:

$$L\left(y_i, \hat{f}(x_i)\right) = \begin{cases} 0 \; y_i = \hat{f}(x_i) \\ 1 \; y_i \neq \hat{f}(x_i) \end{cases}$$

The y-axis in the plot above gives an estimate of the misclassification error rate in the test set. Only one variable is selected according to this analysis.

20.2 Regularized Regression Models

Regularizes involves shrinking the regression model coefficients towards 0 which stabilizes variance in exchange for a small increase in bias. The bet here is that a sparse model is at play with many of the coefficients are zero. The general idea of penalized regression is that the loss function (usually squared error loss) is minimized under a constraint that penalizes for model complexity and/or large absolute values of coefficients [4]. Remember that in the case of OLS (ordinary least squares) regression coefficient estimates are obtained by minimizing:

$$RSS(\beta) = \sum_{i=1}^{N} (y_i - f(x_i))^2$$

$$= \sum_{i=1}^{N} \left(y_i - \beta - \sum_{j=1}^{p} x_{ij}\beta_j \right)^2$$

When there are many predictors the OLS suffers from high variability of the estimated coefficients but having low bias. However, RSS is impacted by both measures of error.

This is where regularized or penalized models help out.

20.2.1 Ridge Regression

The Ridge regression [8,9] for linear regression can be expressed as follows:

$$L_{ridge}\left(\hat{\beta}\right) = \sum_{i=1}^{N} \left(y_i - x_i'\hat{\beta}\right)^2 + \lambda \sum_{i=1}^{N} \hat{\beta}_j^2 = \left\|y - X\hat{\beta}\right\|^2 + \lambda\left\|\hat{\beta}\right\|^2$$

The first term in the expression is the cost term and the second one is the penalty term. The procedure applies the penalty factor λ to the squared norm of the regression coefficients. Ridge regression uses this L_2 penalty (sum of squares of regression coefficients multiplied by the penalty factor), thus shrinking regression coefficients closer to zero [32]. It deals well with highly correlated variables, but does not perform variables selection explicitly (some of variables can remain in the model with coefficient near to 0).

20.2.2 Lasso Regression

Lasso (least absolute shrinkage and selection operator) regression [10] uses L_1 penalty (sum of absolute values of regression coefficients multiplied by the penalty factor), thus allowing for simultaneous variable selection (by forcing some of the coefficients to be exactly zero) and coefficient estimation:

$$L_{lasso}\left(\widehat{\beta}\right) = \sum_{i=1}^{N}\left(y_i - x_i'\widehat{\beta}\right)^2 + \lambda\sum_{i=1}^{N}\left|\widehat{\beta}_j\right|$$

The regression coefficients now cannot be solved analytically and numerical algorithms like coordinate descent are used to find the solutions [7].

Ridge and Lasso process have an important difference about handling multicollinear variables. In Ridge Regression, the coefficients of correlated variables will be similar, while in LASSO, one is usually zeroed and the other retains the full effect. Therefore, Ridge works better when there many covariates of same magnitude of association with the outcome, whereas Lasso works better in a sparse model, that is, when only a small number of predictors are associated with the outcome. Another condition worth noting is that Lasso will pick at most n predictors in the p>>n case and hence further updates to these regularization procedures were made.

20.2.3 Elastic Net Regression

Usually we do not know which case is applicable to us and/or may need to choose a wider number of predictors than Lasso. Therefore, another flexible procedure, Elastic Net [11], has emerged and delivers promising results in most situations where we are interested in variable selection. Elastic net combines L_1 and L_2 penalties with separate penalty factors, thus allowing for subset selection with a better performance in the presence of multicollinearity.

$$\widehat{\beta} = arg \min_{\beta}\|y - X\beta\|^2 + \lambda_2\|\beta\|^2 + \lambda_1\|\beta\|_1$$

We see there are two penalty terms, and setting $\lambda_2 = 0$ gives the Lasso solution, whereas setting $\lambda_1 = 0$ gives the Ridge solution. So, the procedures described earlier are special cases of elastic net. Using both penalties generates a sparse model, and at the same time removes the limitation on # of variables chosen, allows variables to be in a *group (correlated)* and still be chosen and stabilizes the regularization path in difficult structures of data.

20.2.4 Selection of Tuning Parameters

All penalized regression methods require selection of the regularization parameter (hereafter, λ), which determines the strength of the imposed penalty. The most commonly used method to select an optimal value of λ is CV (CV). Usually two values of λ are considered: the value that minimizes the CV mean squared error (MSE) (denoted as λ_{min}) and the maximum value within one standard error from λ_{min} (denoted as λ_{1se}).

In R package 'glmnet', the elastic net family is re-parameterized with a tuning parameter $\alpha \epsilon [0,1]$ to select Ridge, Lasso or somewhere in between (Elastic Net) model selection procedures; in addition, the tuning parameter λ determined the amount of regularization. We will use this package for the examples now. Note that R package 'caret' is another powerful package that allows user even more flexibility in tuning parameter selection through various modes of cross-validation. I leave the exploration of the R package 'caret' to the reader.

I will show how to extract the tuning parameter and the coefficient values at the optimal parameter setting via cross-validation in R package 'glmnet' for our data set with the continuous outcome y.

20.2.5 Variable Selection via R Package 'glmnet'

The R code below reads the data from 'bm.csv', scales the features of the data, and calls glmnet() to perform variable selection for ridge, lasso, and elastic net regularized regressions:

```
>Xy<-cbind(as.data.frame(scale(bm[,3:ncol(bm)])), safe=bm$y)
>colnames(Xy)[ncol(Xy)]='y';
>par(mfrow=c(1,3))
>fit.ridge=glmnet(y=Xy[,13], x=as.matrix(Xy[,1:12]),alpha=0)
>plot_glmnet(fit.ridge, label=TRUE, xvar="dev")
>fit.lasso=glmnet(y=Xy[,13], x=as.matrix(Xy[,1:12]),alpha=1)
>plot_glmnet(fit.lasso, label=TRUE, xvar="dev")
>fit.enet=glmnet(y=Xy[,13], x=as.matrix(Xy[,1:12]),alpha=.5)
>plot_glmnet(fit.enet, label=TRUE, xvar="dev")
```

The plots produce the results of the fit side-by-side. The same variables are being chosen by regularization as our earlier analysis of best subset selection: feat3 and feat4. Note the parameter alpha chooses whether we are fitting the Ridge, Lasso, or the Elastic Net model (Figure 20.3).

As you can see, the left plot showing ridge regression fits, the coefficients do not reach 0; however, in Lasso and Elastic net, several variable coefficients remain 0. I plotted fraction of deviance explained but could have easily plotted the tuning parameter on the x-axis.

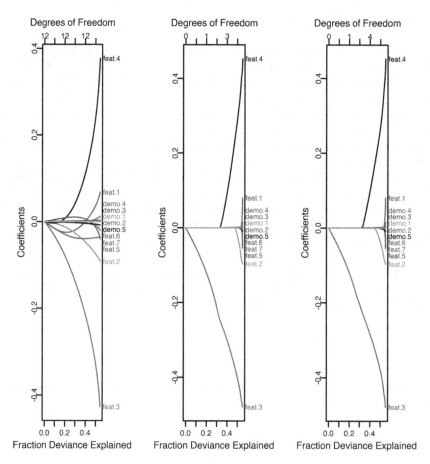

FIGURE 20.3
Ridge, Lasso and Elastic Net variable selection results.

Now let us show how we get the optimal tuning parameter value through CV; we will plot the value of the CV with tuning parameter (lambda) values on the x-axis. Note we use the ridge regression (alpha=0) model for this example.

```
>cvfit=cv.glmnet(x=as.matrix(Xy[,1:12]),y=Xy[,13],type.measure
="mse",alpha=0,nfolds=10)
>plot(cvfit)
>log(cvfit$lambda.1se)
[1] -1.421166
> coef(cvfit,s="lambda.1se")
```

```
(Intercept)    0.364
feat.1        -0.006
feat.2        -0.042
feat.3        -0.193
feat.4         0.090
feat.5         0.008
feat.6        -0.002
feat.7        -0.039
demo.1         0.002
demo.2         0.001
demo.3         0.002
demo.4         0.000
demo.5        -0.004
```

The parameter s is the model size at the optimal lambda where the MSE is minimized.

We see that feat3 and feat4 have coefficients with largest magnitude.

The plot of the cross-validated fit looks like that in Figure 20.4. The plot matches the optimal value of the tuning parameter lambda.

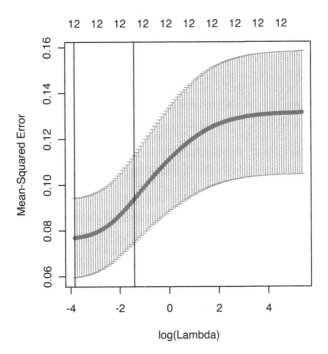

FIGURE 20.4
Tuning parameter selection in Ridge Regression.

Note, I have stayed with R packages bestglm and glmnet through this chapter because I wanted to do variable selection using information criteria (older methods), as well as regularization or shrinkage (newer methods) on the same data with relatively few biomarkers. If you are investigating more than a dozen or so biomarkers and clinical factors in the regression setting and you are approaching the p>>n scenario, I recommend proceeding directly with shrinkage methods or other learning methods suitable for high-dimensional variable selection. The reader can check out the **'caret'** package for various newer machine learning methods for data sets containing many biomarkers.

20.3 Regularization with Interaction Effects

In this chapter, I have introduced the general Lasso regularization procedure in the regression setting. There are many variations of Lasso in the statistical learning literature. As data complexity has grown, these procedures have given rise to more varieties that are suited for the data.

Since our goal may very well be to build a model between the clinical outcome and biomarker by treatment interaction, I want to introduce a synthetic data set that contains the treatment variable; and a procedure that considers all first-order (pair-wise) interactions for continuous or categorical covariates. Again, there are various methods that will perform variable selection including interaction effects using regularization; however, I will mention one such procedure to give the reader a flavor of the problem and a solution for biomarker analysis.

The learning of interactions via the *hierarchical-group Lasso* was proposed by Lim and Hastie [12]. The authors refer to a group analogue to the Lasso, called the group-Lasso [13], which sets groups of variables to zero. The idea behind Lim's method is to set up main effects and interactions as groups and then perform variable selection via the group-Lasso. Since there will be $p + \binom{p}{2}$ predictors and pairwise interactions, the problem might be computationally infeasible to solve for moderate or large p. For small p (which is close to our scenario of a few biomarkers), group-Lasso is fit through all the groups, otherwise a screening is performed first to filter the predictors. The methodology is discussed by Lim in their paper. Note that the strict hierarchical nature of the main effects and interactions, where both main effects have to be present in order for the interaction to be present, is preserved in this method.

20.3.1 Data Set

The data set Xy contains the data set in bmtrt.csv, which includes a column for treatment

```
> head(Xy)
       BM_1        BM_2       BM_3       BM_4       BM_5       BM_6
1 -0.73922011 -0.2213106  0.2103968  2.0337030 -4.012667 -1.7736200
2  1.03192696  1.6611258 -0.7225904 -1.4187845 -5.073719  0.8758690
3 -0.90234757 -0.1538720 -1.1278491 -0.2027323 -4.288533  0.1619535
4  0.04287871  0.1209942  0.2352843 -0.4705628 -6.278969 -1.1970587
5 -1.93689044 -2.6522463 -1.3414828  0.3541399 -6.199020 -1.7438352
6  2.21876339  1.9974832 -0.1225671  0.3323039 -6.700173  0.5756311
       BM_7        BM_8       BM_9       BM_10     trt        y
1  1.1327296   0.95354795  1.2659156 -0.33653774   0   9.096544
2 -0.3980706   0.03406953 -0.7527621 -1.07206095   0  10.329784
3 -0.9197886  -0.48814111  0.4131020 -0.09884493   0  10.877213
4  0.1918441   0.70375804 -1.4088384 -2.20081885   0   7.350952
5 -1.4310876   0.30585219 -0.4298816 -1.93589767   0   9.206562
6 -0.9786918  -0.95302318 -1.3048736 -2.38772695   0  10.484881
```

It is a synthetic data set that has 100 rows (one row per patient) and the treatment (trt) is split 1:1 to control and drug regimen. The response variable y is a continuous variable.

20.3.2 Learning Interactions via R Package 'glinternet'

```
>library(glinternet)
>set.seed(617)

>num.biom=10    # number of biomarkers
>Xy=read.csv("bmtrt.csv")
>Xy=data.frame(scale(Xy[,3:ncol(Xy)]),y=Xy[,2])
>X=Xy[,c(1:(num.biom+1))]
>y=Xy$y

>cv_fit <- glinternet.cv(X, y,numLevels=c(rep(1,num.biom),2))
>plot(cv_fit)
```

It is very simply to fit the glinternet model via CV using the R package [14]. However, we do have to extract the coefficients to make sense of what has been learned.

Peter Straka's website [15] provides a useful tutorial of this package and makes the coefficient extraction more user-friendly. Figure 20.5 is the output of the CV procedure following Peter's code. The plot above shows the MSE plotted against the regularization parameter, lambda.

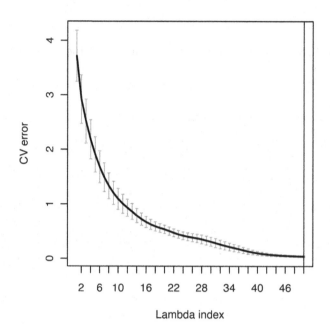

FIGURE 20.5
Cross-validation error vs tuning parameter.

Using the following command, as suggested by Peter, we choose lambda to be optimal conservatively, that is, when the CV error is below the minimum plus one standard deviation. The reasoning is that choosing the λ corresponding to the minimum value of MSE may not result into a sufficiently regularized model. Hence empirical studies recommend selecting a λ, which is the largest value of λ within one standard error of minimum MSE value at the minimum λ.

```
> i_1Std <- which(cv_fit$lambdaHat1Std == cv_fit$lambda)
> i_1Std
[1] 46
```

The glinternet procedure reports the main effects and interaction terms it has chosen after the regularization process has worked on the data. As shown, the lambda parameter to be used is 46.

```
##Which categorical variable is chosen
> names(NL)[idx_cat[coefs$mainEffects$cat]]
[1] "trt"

##Which continuous variable is chosen
> names(NL)[idx_num[coefs$mainEffects$cont]]
[1] "BM_1" "BM_6" "BM_8" "BM_9" "BM_2" "BM_3" "BM_5" "BM_7" "BM_10"
```

The categorical variable 'trt' (treatment variable) and biomarkers 1, 2, 3, 6, 7, 8, 9, and 10 have been chosen as main effects.

```
>coefs <- coef(cv_fit$glinternetFit)[[i_1Std]]
>coefs$mainEffects
>coefs$interactions
$catcat
NULL

$contcont
     [,1] [,2]
[1,]    1    2
[2,]    1    3
[3,]    2    8
[4,]    3    9
[5,]    5    6
[6,]    5    8
[7,]    6    7
[8,]    9   10

$catcont
     [,1] [,2]
[1,]    1    1
[2,]    1    2
[3,]    1    3
[4,]    1    5
[5,]    1    6
[6,]    1    7
[7,]    1    9
```

The continuous–continuous interactions learned were BM1-BM2, BM1-BM3, and so on.

The categorical–continuous interactions learned were trt-BM1, trt-BM2, and so on.

Another wonderful snippet pointed out in Peter's website is to check the MSE of the final learned model and compare it to regular Lasso:

```
#Model from glinternet
> sqrt(cv_fit$cvErr[[i_1Std]])
[1] 0.2289548

#Model from regular Lasso regression via cross-validation
> X1 <- model.matrix(y ~ . - 1, Xy)
> cv_glmnet <- cv.glmnet(X1,y)
> sqrt(min(cv_glmnet$cvm))
[1] 0.7960467
```

We see that a smaller MSE is achieved from the optimal model obtained from glinternet.

20.3.3 Penalized Coefficients and Prediction

Once we have run the glinternet() procedure, we will want to extract the final coefficients for the optimal λ. The coefficient vector (beta vector) is stored in the variable 'coefs'. Note some of the interactions and main effects have been shrunk to exactly 0 and do not appear in 'coefs'. We will compare it with regression coefficients of OLS model containing the same set of main effects and first-order interactions.

Table 20.2 shows the side-by-side comparison between OLS and Lasso via glinternet of only those coefficients chosen by Lasso via glinternet.

We see the coefficients are quite different. The Lasso estimate of 'trt' or treatment main effect is more accurate, since the data were simulated with a difference of 5 in the means of treated and placebo groups. It is important to

TABLE 20.2

OLS vs LASSO – regression coefficients

Term	Lasso -glinternet	OLS
Intercept	2.142404	8.367746882
trt	−4.081159	−6.357940842
BM1	1.045107	0.930953075
BM6	0.1456438	0.310451078
BM8	−0.2259992	−0.180845678
BM9	0.5127078	1.060565609
BM2	−0.1255591	−0.241346962
BM3	−0.5079127	−1.310907017
BM5	−0.1711581	−0.21247433
BM7	−0.329564	−0.058482477
BM10	0.0103989	0.005037727
trt:BM1	0.09760292	0.521369043
trt:BM2	0.1505555	0.282947059
trt:BM3	0.5595303	1.388939512
trt:BM5	−0.1742341	−0.392618069
trt:BM6	−0.0533937	−0.21107443
trt:BM7	−0.3220891	−0.824317994
trt:BM9	−0.1760885	−0.76088893
BM1: BM2	0.01876656	0.02447576
BM1: BM3	0.0028189	0.004509848
BM2: BM8	−0.0055082	−0.003365655
BM3: BM9	0.00810164	0.01401464
BM5: BM6	0.00731535	0.010209558
BM5: BM8	−0.0084025	−0.019679431
BM6:BM7	−0.0231812	−0.017693883
BM9: BM10	0.01156015	0.009843549

note that Lasso and other penalized methods introduce a small amount of controlled bias, in exchange of making the variability of the estimates more stable. Therefore, the penalized coefficients give rise to a prediction model that is more stable across test sets of unseen data.

Prediction is very simple regardless of the Lasso model you use. The ordinary Lasso and the group Lasso for interaction effect glinternet have been discussed here.

Let us split the biomarker data with treatment into a training set of 140 subjects and a test set of 60 subjects. I used more subjects to train, since there are main and interaction effects and the number of subjects is small.

The splitting of data into training and test is being done twice, once inside the call of glinternet to choose λ in CV in the data set with 140 subjects, next we use the remaining test set of 60 subjects to predict the response variable y.

```
> train=sample (200 ,140)
> cv_fit2 <- glinternet.cv(Xy[train,c(1:11)],
             Xy[train,12],numLevels=c(rep(1,num.biom),2))
> mean((Xy[-train,12] -predict (cv_fit2 ,Xy[-train,-12]))^2)
[1] 0.09766074
```

Lastly, the R package 'caret' allows the statistician to nest both estimation and prediction inside CV loops. It is a premium R package containing the most common and popular implementation of Lasso and other regularization procedures through versatile implementation of CV. At the time of writing this book, there were more than 200 models available in 'caret', even though glinternet() is not one of them [17].

21

Tree-Based Models

Many of the statistical learning models are rooted in probability theory, yet decision trees are known for their ability to mimic human decision-making. In fact, clinicians find this type of data representation particularly intuitive and interpretable. By human decision-making, I mean if–then–else decision-making criteria based on logic. A decision *tree* is a *tree*-like procedure of decisions and their application is in many fields of data science. The tree of decision-making marks a path from 'root' (at the top) to the bottommost 'leaves' (at the bottom), where each new observation for prediction will traverse the path and ultimately gets binned into one of the leaves. Classification and regression trees (CARTs) as established by Breiman et al. [25] are a popular method for predicting outcomes, where a recursive partitioning method was used to build classification (binary outcome) and regression trees (continuous outcome). The algorithm works by recursively splitting the feature or variable space into a set of non-overlapping regions and predicting the most likely value of the dependent outcome within each region.

A tree represents a set of nested logical if–then conditions on the values of the features variables that allows for the prediction of the value of the dependent variable based on the observed values of the feature variables. CART can handle missing values. The model can be tested on a separately specified test set (independent validation set). Additionally, the tree can be saved and used subsequently on additional test sets.

21.1 Regression Tree

The procedure

- Starts with a single split or region R_1 and loop as follows
- Selects a region R_m based on a single predictor X_1, and a split or cut-point c, where splitting R_m with the criterion $X_j < c$ produces the largest drop in RSS:

$$\sum_{m=1}^{|T|} \sum_{x_i \in R_m} \left(y_i - \bar{y}_{R_m} \right)^2$$

- Ends looping where there are fewer than, say, 5 observations in each region.

This procedure grows the full tree from the root (in top) toward the leaves (in bottom).

Obviously, this is different from ordinary least squares (OLS) regression, where we have model for $E(Y|X)$, where Y is continuous and X are predictors. In trees we are partitioning, the feature (data) space (X) into different regions and taking means of y in the divided feature regions. The usual parameters for regression-like coefficients, P values, R^2 of OLS are not present in the regression tree. Regression trees are nonparametric and nonlinear; you can use tree to model non-normal data and as mentioned before the splits in feature space may be very human interpretable. So, each method has its advantages.

Let us apply the regression tree building procedure offered in the R package 'rpart' [25] to the biomarker data with treatment variable contained in bmtrt.csv. Therneau et al. have implemented many of the ideas for CART book and programs of Breiman, Friedman, Olshen, and Stone [25] in this useful R package.

21.1.1 Why Use Regression Trees and Not Linear Regression?

Before we apply the procedure to data, it is worth mentioning when we are likely to use regression modeling vs regression trees. Least squares regression models are built on strong assumptions: Gaussian distribution of the outcome variable Y; predictors having additive effect on Y; homoscedasticity; and so on. Importantly, linear regression model builds a global model on the enter feature space for Y using a single formula. This scenario can get more complex with many variables (p>>n) and numerous nonlinear interactions between variables in the large global space of **X**. Nevertheless, linear regression with its ability to handle interactions and polynomials is a very strong methodology for estimation of the underlying relationship you are not in very high dimension.

Regression trees on the other hand are nonparametric procedures that use divide-and-conquer strategy on the feature space to predict y. At each step, it is trying to do the best split based on the local level of information available, where the interactions of variables are easier seen than on the global level. The simple model at each leaf is the average of y values at that leaf. Trees do not guarantee having reached a global optimal for cost complexity however.

Which one to use depends on (i) the data you have at hand and (ii) what the objectives are of your analysis.

In the context of biomarkers, you have to answer whether you are trying to achieve a 'cutpoint' approach with your multiple biomarkers (e.g., responders are those with $X >$ cut1 AND $Y >$ cut2) or a weighted combination approach where the composite biomarker is a function of other biomarkers (e.g., c= a*X + b*Y)?

Regression trees certainly give a very simple, interpretable model, and is well-suited for prediction. It also is agnostic about parametric assumption of associations between Y and X. It is good to have both tools available for modeling. If you are interested in variable selection and prediction, you will most likely rely on regularized regression methods or pruned trees to siphon out the most important variables. It is best to compare the results of both the regularized linear regressions and regression trees with respect to RSS to determine which model did better.

21.1.2 Regression Tree Building Using R Package 'rpart'

First, we use the whole data set to build a regression tree using 'rpart'. We then use the plot function to display the tree.

```
> library(rpart)           # Popular decision tree algorithm
> library(rpart.plot)

> tree.bm = rpart(y~.,data=Xy)
> rpart.plot(tree.bm)
```

The output has clearly chosen treatment (trt) as the first variable to split on when modeling the variability of continuous outcome variable y (Figure 21.1).

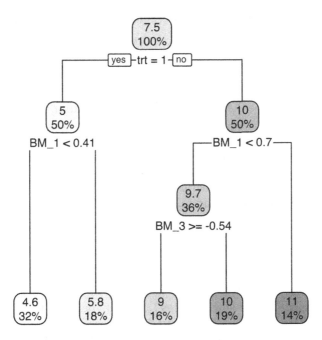

FIGURE 21.1
Regression Tree.

The tree shows that 50% of the observations were treated and the other 50% were not; the mean of the outcome variable y was 5 in the treated group and 10 in the untreated group. This agrees with the 'truth', since the data is synthetically created from pre-set parameters that match those estimated by the tree.

21.1.2.1 Minimal Cost-Complexity Pruning

How do we control overfitting in building the regression tree? Finding the optimal subtree by cross-validation is not possible (because the problem is even harder than best subset selection)! We stop growing tree when the RSS does not drop more than a threshold with any more splits. The procedure commonly used is the *minimal cost-complexity pruning*, where growing the tree is controlled by a parameter called CP (complexity parameter) in the algorithm. The commands printcp() and plot() of the rpart object 'tree.bm' above will give descriptive and visual summary of the CP. The more splitting that occurs, the deeper the tree, the more overfitting, and we are back to the bias-variance tradeoff paradigm. Pruning is a tool available to prevent overfitting in trees.

Even before pruning, there are three general parameters that are used to limit growing the tree:

- Minbucket: no. of observations in a terminal node cannot be less than this parameter value (say 5). This prevents too fine splitting of the data
- Minsplit: no. of observations in a node before permitting the node to be split
- Maxdepth: maximum depth of the tree (from root to leaf)

The user is free to set these to control the tree-building process. They are selectable from the rpart function with the control parameter.

The tree is built and then pruned to prevent overfitting by minimizing this function $Min_T \sum_{m=1}^{|T|} \sum_{x_i \in R_m} (y_i - \bar{y}_{R_m})^2 + \alpha |T|$

where the total cost of the tree, which is a combination of the variance and the tree size, times a penalty factor $\alpha \geq 0$. If $\alpha = 0$, then we have the full tree. As α grows, we penalize the addition of nodes to the tree. If $\alpha = \infty$, then we select no splits or the null tree.

How do we choose α through cross-validation?

- Split the training set into 10 folds.
- For k = 1, ..., 10, using every fold except the kth:
  - Construct a sequence of trees $T_1, ..., T_m$ (where m= # of predictors) for a range of values of α, and find the prediction for each region (remember a tree is a collection of regions) in each one.

- For each tree T_i' calculate the RSS on the test set using the prediction for each region calculated above.
- Select the parameter α that minimizes the average test error.

We can visualize a two-way table of α and T_is at the end of the process, which makes it easier to choose the α and the corresponding minimum T_i.

NOTE: We are doing all fitting, including the construction of the trees, using only the training data.

Note that 'rpart' by default will use cross-validation to choose the optimal complexity parameter, whereas the 'tree' package' does not (you will need to use 'cv.tree' and other functions if you are using the 'tree' package). Plotting the complexity parameter (CP) values against the cross-validated error calculated by the 'rpart' algorithm. Clearly, the most important node (trt) has the biggest RSS drop in the tree building process (Figure 21.2).

We can extract the value of minimum CP, which is returned as 0.01. When we print the tree at the optimal CP value, we are given the same as the tree from above (Figure 21.3).

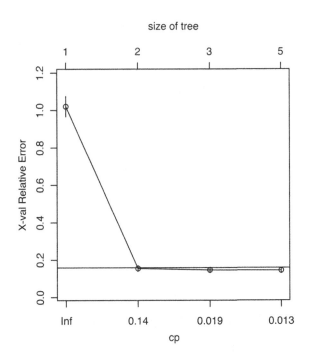

FIGURE 21.2
Cost Complexity Parameter (CP) of Regression Tree vs Relative Error.

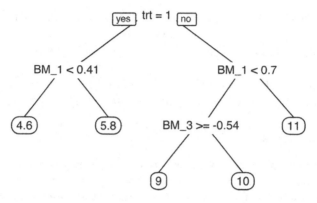

FIGURE 21.3
Regression Tree at Optimal CP.

```
# find best value of cp
min_cp =
tree.bm$cptable[which.min(tree.bm$cptable[,"xerror"]),"CP"]
min_cp
# prune tree using best cp
tree.bm.prune = prune(tree.bm, cp = min_cp)
prp(tree.bm.prune)
```

This means that rpart had returned the best pruned tree in the first step for
this data set.

21.2 Classification Tree

Classification trees work the same way as regression trees, except that outcome is binary or categorical. And instead of RSS, the procedure predicts the
response by majority vote, that is, pick the most common class in every region.

The R code, where we simply cut the outcome variable at median to generate a binary outcome, is given as follows (Figure 21.4):

```
> resp=ifelse(y<median(y),0,1)

> Xy=cbind(Xy[1:11],resp)
> tree.bm=rpart(resp~.,data=Xy)
> rpart.plot(tree.bm)
# find best value of cp
> min_cp =
tree.bm$cptable[which.min(tree.bm$cptable[,"xerror"]),"CP"]
# prune tree using best cp
> tree.bm.prune = prune(tree.bm, cp = min_cp)
> rpart.plot(tree.bm.prune)
```

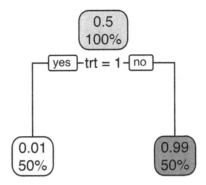

FIGURE 21.4
Classification Tree.

We see that in the left leaf node, we have half the observations; and in the right leaf node, the other half. The predicted probability of each class is also reported in each node, where 99% of the events are predicted to be in the branch where the patients were not treated.

21.3 Other Trees

The R package 'rpart' supports trees for various types of data including classification, ANOVA, Poisson, and exponential. Also, note that you can build trees for multiclass outcome variables with 'rpart', which is very useful, as you may have an outcome, which separates patients into low, moderate, and high categories, for example. The reader can explore this package on how to build trees through recursion for various types of data.

21.3.1 Survival Trees

Survival data is an area of active research for building trees and forests. The evolution of the methodological research is captured in the review by Bou-Hamad et al. [29].

One of the recent packages that implement survival regression trees is 'LTRCtrees' [30]. Let us discuss this R package a bit here. The *LTRCtrees* package fits survival trees for left-truncated and right censored (LTRC) data, as well as interval-censored survival data. For right censored data, the tree algorithms present in R packages 'rpart' and 'partykit' are used to fit a survival tree. The *LTRCtrees* package extends the survival tree algorithms in these two packages to fit trees for LTRC data, as well as interval-censored survival data. The package also accommodates survival trees for data with time-varying covariates.

Before we use this package, let us choose the biomarker data set given in the R package 'bhm' [31–33]. The package 'bhm' fits Bayesian hierarchical models for predictive and prognostic biomarker effects with binary data and survival data with an unknown biomarker cutoff point. So, we can compare the splits of biomarker derived by the 'LTRCTrees' package, as well as the 'bhm' package.

Keep in mind that this example data set below given in the 'bhm' package only has a single biomarker, but still I am using it for illustrative purposes of constructing trees for survival data with biomarker and treatment covariates.

```
#Survival data
##
## Generate a random data set
n = 300
b = c(0.5, 1, 1.5)
data = surv.gendat(n, c0 = 0.40, beta = b)
age = runif(n, 0, 1)*100
tm = data[, 1]
status = data[, 2]
trt = data[, 3]
ki67 = data[, 4]


## fit a biomarker threshold survival model with one single
cut point
fit = bhm(Surv(tm, status)~ki67+trt+age, interaction = TRUE,
B=5, R=10)
##Now use LTRCART
library(LTRCtrees)
DATA=data.frame(tm,status,ki67,trt,age)
DATA$t0=rep(0,nrow(DATA))
set.seed(650)
idx=sample(seq(1:nrow(DATA)),100,replace = FALSE)
Train=DATA[idx,]
Test=DATA[!idx,]

LTRCART.obj <- LTRCART(Surv(t0,tm, status)
~ ki67+trt+age, Train)
LTRCIT.obj <- LTRCIT(Surv(t0,tm, status)
~ ki67+trt+age, Train)

rpart.plot.version1(LTRCART.obj)
```

First, the results of finding the optimal cutpoint for biomarker ki67 derived from the Bayesian model in 'bhm' is:

```
ki67 biomarker threshold:
                Estimate    2.5%      97.5%
     55.23264%  0.4033      0.3971    0.429
```

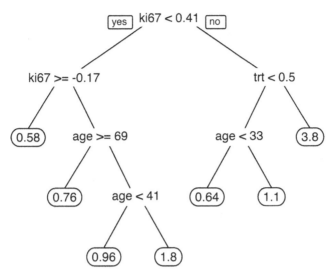

FIGURE 21.5
Survival Tree.

And now let us look at where the tree method in 'LTRCtrees' splits the bio-marker using the optimal pruning algorithm (Figure 21.5).

We see that the biomarker is pretty much split at the root node at the same cutpoint as the Bayesian method for selecting biomarkers.

21.3.2 Random Forest

CART pruning is sufficient for addressing overfitting in trees in the low-dimensional setting we have discussed with biomarkers. However, if you are in the realm of investigating 25 or more features (biomarkers or other clinical factors), or there are many complex interactions of your features, you need to use methods well suited for higher dimensions like the random forest. In this case, hundreds of trees are built and averaged to get a very low predictor error. This is called *ensemble learning*. You can also use Random Forest in low-dimensional cases, but you would not get much more information than CART regression or classification trees since the complexity of information is low. You can learn a lot about Random Forest from Breiman et al. [27] and use the R package 'caret' [28] to implement it on your data set.

22

Cluster Analysis

Unsupervised learning is where you only have input data (X), which are the covariates and no corresponding labels (outcome variable or Y). Simply put, the goal for unsupervised learning is to model the underlying structure or distribution in the data in order to learn more about the data. This is a topic that comes up less frequently in the context of drug development where we usually focus on finding predictive biomarkers or surrogate endpoints. If the statistician who is working on drug development is interested in finding clusters of prognostic markers, which stand for disease heterogeneity or severity, for example, then the statistician can run clustering procedures.

With the outcome variable omitted or not identified, the algorithm finds the underlying group or structure in the predictor (feature) space of the data set. For example, for a gene expression data of diverse types of tumors in patients present in a data set, where the columns are patients and rows are the genes, we expect the patients with similar tumor type (w.r.t. gene expression profiles) to cluster together based on their gene expression values.

Clustering is but one unsupervised method that we cover in this chapter. The topic of unsupervised methods is vast and I encourage the reader to research this topic in detail if undertaking unsupervised exploration of data. I cover the topic of clustering very briefly in this chapter. For cluster analysis, I recommend the tutorial at STHDA [34], which provides a quick start with R in clustering. In addition, the R library 'cluster' [36] is a good introductory collection of functions to do cluster analysis.

Clustering analysis methods described here are best suited for small datasets. With huge number of predictors, advanced methods would be necessary to group the data.

22.1 k-Means and PAM Clustering

The first step is to decide on a metric of importance in clustering, which is the *measure of dissimilarity* between clusters; we want this metric to be high and the within-clusters distance to be low. This metric is often the Euclidean, Manhattan, or Mahalanobis distance.

The second step is to choose the clustering method. Three of the popular procedures for clustering are (i) k-means clustering, (ii) PAM clustering, which stands for Partition around medoids, and (iii) hierarchical clustering.

The k-means algorithm is parameterized by the value k, which is the number of clusters that you want to create. This is a classical algorithm that constructs a partition by computing k centroids minimizing the overall intracluster dissimilarity.

The algorithm begins by creating k centroids. It then iterates between an assign step (where each sample is assigned to its closest centroid) and an update step (where each centroid is updated to become the mean of all the samples that are assigned to it). This iteration continues until some stopping criteria is met; for example, if no sample is reassigned to a different centroid.

The k-means algorithm makes the assumptions that the data can be separated into spheres; that all variables have the same variance and that each cluster has roughly equal number of observations.

PAM clustering is similar to k-means algorithm except it works on medoids and hence more robust to outliers. The PAM algorithm searches for k representative objects in a data set formed by k medoids and then assigns each object to the closest medoid in order to create clusters. Its aim is to minimize the sum of dissimilarities between the objects in a cluster and the center of the same cluster (medoid). It is known to be a robust version of k-means as it is considered to be less sensitive to outliers.

Agglomerative hierarchical clustering, instead, builds clusters incrementally, producing a tree or dendrogram. This algorithm begins by assigning each sample to its own cluster (top level). At each step, the two clusters that are the most similar are merged; the algorithm continues until all of the clusters have been merged. Unlike k-means, you do not need to specify a k parameter: once the dendrogram has been produced, you can navigate the layers of the tree to see which number of clusters makes the most sense to your particular application.

22.1.1 R Code for PAM Clustering

Let us look at an example provided in the website above [34] for PAM clustering.

```
#Clustering
library(stats)
library(cluster)
library(NbClust)
library(mclust)
library(cluster)
library(clValid)
library("cluster")
pam.res <- pam(my_data, 3)
```

```
#Get only the predictors
x=Xy[,1:11]
corr<-cor(x, method = c("spearman"))
heatmap(x = corr)
my_data=data.frame(scale(x[,1:10]),x[,11])
library("factoextra")

#compute k-means
fviz_nbclust(my_data, kmeans, method = "gap_stat")

km.res <- kmeans(my_data, 2, nstart = 10)
fviz_cluster(km.res,data=my_data,geom="point")

# Compute PAM
library("cluster")
pam.res <- pam(my_data, 3)
# Visualize
fviz_cluster(pam.res,geom="point")# Compute
hierarchical clustering
```

The optimal # of clusters identified by kmeans is 2 (Figure 22.1).

With both kmeans and PAM, you can use the algorithm to determine the optimum number of clusters. For determination of number of clusters, I recommend looking at the R package 'factoextra' and the function fviz_nbclust [35] and the R package 'cluster' [36].

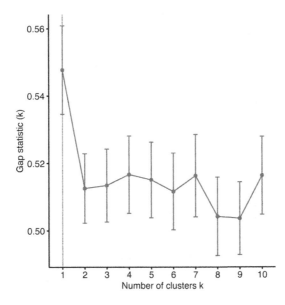

FIGURE 22.1
Optimal number of clusters.

22.2 Hierarchical Clustering

Hierarchical clustering is another powerful approach to partition clusters for identifying groups in the data set. It is often used to cluster life sciences data that often has hierarchy built-in. Hierarchical clustering has the distinct advantage that any valid measure of distance can be used. In fact, the observations themselves are not required: all that is used is a matrix of distances. It does not require one to prespecify the number of clusters. The result of hierarchical clustering is a tree-based representation of the objects, which is known as *dendrogram*. Observations can be subdivided into groups by cutting the dendrogram at a desired similarity level resulting into a user-chosen number of clusters. A popular way of doing cluster analysis is to determine k=the # of cluster through PAM or k means and then using Hierarchical Clustering to group the data matrix columns into k clusters.

A third step is involved in hierarchical clustering, which is the selection of linkage methods for agglomeration of the clusters. The most common types of methods are as follows:

- Maximum or complete linkage clustering: It computes all pairwise dissimilarities between the elements in cluster 1 and the elements in cluster 2, and considers the largest value of these dissimilarities as the distance between the two clusters. It tends to produce more compact clusters.

- Minimum or single linkage clustering: It computes all pairwise dissimilarities between the elements in cluster 1 and the elements in cluster 2 and considers the smallest of these dissimilarities as a linkage criterion. It tends to produce long, 'loose' clusters.

- Mean or average linkage clustering: It computes all pairwise dissimilarities between the elements in cluster 1 and the elements in cluster 2 and considers the average of these dissimilarities as the distance between the two clusters.

- Centroid linkage clustering: It computes the dissimilarity between the centroid for cluster 1 and the centroid for cluster 2.

- Ward's minimum variance method: It minimizes the total within-cluster variance. At each step, the pair of clusters with minimum between-cluster distance are merged.

22.2.1 R Code for Hierarchical Clustering

Typically the Ward's methods gives a very good clustering of biomarker data.

```
#compute hierarchical
res.hc <- my_data %>%
```

```
scale() %>%                          # Scale the data
dist(method = "euclidean") %>% # Compute dissimilarity
                                       matrix
hclust(method = "ward.D2")       # Compute hierachical
                                     clustering

# Visualize using factoextra
# Cut in 2 groups and color by groups
D=fviz_dend(res.hc, k = 2, # Cut in four groups
        cex = 0.5, # label size
        k_colors = c("#2E9FDF", "#00AFBB"),
        color_labels_by_k = TRUE, # color labels by groups
        rect = TRUE # Add rectangle around groups

)

#Extract info from the dendrogram
dend.data=attr(F,"dendrogram")
table(my_data[,11],km.res$cluster)   #compare to the treatment
variable
```

The dendrogram is plotted with >*plot(D)* as shown in Figure 22.2.

For more insight into cluster analysis, including cluster validation and advanced clustering methods, you may find the book by Kassambra [36] useful to read. In addition, for a quick starter on Hierarchical Cluster Analysis, refer to the online resources in GitHub [37].

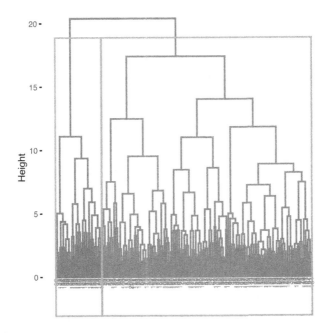

FIGURE 22.2
Cluster dendrogram.

23

Graphical Models

Network analysis is a relatively novel approach to identify possible bio-marker-related mechanisms in a disease being modulated by treatment. It is important to know how to interpret the visual representation of the network, as well as to control for overfitting the model.

It is useful to conceptualize several components of network analysis as described below:

- *Graphical Representation*: The network is a graphical representation of nodes and edges. Nodes are represented as variables (e.g., biomarkers, treatment, clinical factors, outcome variables, etc.) and edges are statistical parameters (e.g., correlation, partial correlation, covariance, etc.).

- *Multivariate Data*: The analysis accommodates the simultaneous modeling of all variables by the matrix of multivariate data, such as pairwise partial correlations. There is no delineation between a predictor and explanatory variables in network analysis, as in regression. Identifying significant partial correlations between variables X and Y indicates there may be an association between them, after adjusting for linear dependence on all other variables in the model.

- *Plotting Algorithm*: There are several plotting algorithms for the network graph. One such algorithm is the Fruchterman–Reingold (FR) algorithm [17], commonly used in network analysis. This is a force-directed graph method [18], which creates a graph of balls connected by strings. The ball are the nodes, and the strings are the edges (statistical parameters). The goal is to position the balls in a way they do not overlap each other for ease of viewing. No positional (spatial) interpretation can be made from the graph about the circles (nodes). For more information on visualizing different types of multivariate data, see the tutorial by Johansson et al. [19].

- *Variable Selection*: As in previous chapters on regularization of regression models, the network of partial correlations can also be penalized for variable selection with respect to the edges. In the end, we are able to detect a sparse network with only the true inter-relationship highlighted in the graph network.

The components of network analysis make it very useful in any of the following scenarios:

- analyzing data sets with smaller sample sizes and many covariates (p>>n)
- when the biomarkers or efficacy (biomarkers, endpoints or others) are not known in terms of hierarchy or relative importance
- when the interrelationship between the variables need to be understood
- variable selection is needed so that conditionally independent relationships between the variables are retained and the spurious ones disappear

For these reasons, network analysis could add significant value to analyzing data when a new therapeutic area is being studied with the help of many variables collected from the patient. Estimating the interconnectedness between variables and regularizing the network topology in order to detect significant associations is a type of exploration which remains underutilized in biomarker research.

Note the graphs we will generate in this book are undirected. We make no assumptions of latent variables in the model; therefore, no causal relationship will be assumed to exist between variables. We limit our attention to detecting association between variables in our graphical models (causal or not) after adjusting for all other variables.

23.1 Partial Correlation Network

Partial correlation is a statistical tool used to perform network analysis of multivariate data. In psychology, latent class variables have been traditionally modeled via structural equation modeling for a long time. In other fields, we have been more familiar with a similar idea from the Gaussian Graphical Models (GGMs), which provides a way to estimate the variance–covariance matrix of the data arising from n-dimensional multivariate normal distribution. The dimension of the variance–covariance matrix (or the inverse or precision matrix) is p × p when there are p variables under study. The idea is to model the pairwise association between each variable. The partial correlation has been suggested which is defined as the conditional correlation between variables X and Y, given the remaining variables [20,21]. Once the partial correlation parameters are estimated, we can visualize the matrix in various ways.

One popular way is to create a heatmap; another informative way is to display via graphical models. The R package 'igraph' is one of the libraries that facilitate the visualization of the inter-relationships between the covariates.

As an example, we use the data set with biomarkers (BMs), treatment variable (trt), and continuous outcome (y) presented in Chapter 2. We then work toward building a graph of the partial correlation network of the data in the following steps.

- Step 1: We create the variance–covariance matrix by modeling the pairwise partial correlation between all the variables. Partial correlation is the correlation between X and Y when the linear effect of correlation of all other variables have been removed.

- Step 2: We set the nodes of the graph as the covariates; and the edges as the pairwise partial correlations. If an edge does not exist between X and Y, it means that these two are independent of each other, given all the other variables in the model.

- Step 3: We plot the graphical representation of the model estimated parameters with the condition that an edge will be plotted only if the partial correlation is above absolute 0.3. This condition simply allows you to see fewer edges.

23.1.1 Plotting Graphical Models of Partial Correlation via R

The R library 'igraph' plots the adjacency matrix of the graph from the variance–covariance matrix; and the R library 'ppcor' forms the edges of the variance–covariance matrix as the partial correlation between each pair of variables (Figure 23.1).

```
> library(igraph)
> library(ppcor)
> cor_mat=pcor(Xy)$estimate
> cor_mat<-as.matrix(cor_mat)
> diag(cor_mat) <- 0

> cor_g <- graph_from_adjacency_matrix(cor_mat,
  mode='undirected',
  weighted="pcor")

> cor_edge_list <- as_data_frame(cor_g, 'edges')
> only_sig <- cor_edge_list[abs(cor_edge_list$pcor) > .3, ]
> new_g <- graph_from_data_frame(only_sig, directed=FALSE)
> plot(new_g)
```

The graph above shows very similar results to those obtained in Chapter 2 using regularized regression model 'glinternet'. But since we modeled many

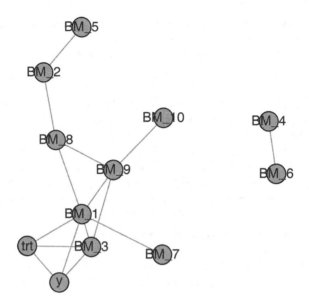

FIGURE 23.1
Partial Correlation Network.

pairwise relationships, we need to account for multiple comparisons in our graphical model. Regularization techniques like LASSO from regression models are available for graphical models as well. I cover that topic in Section V.

23.1.2 Regularization of Networks via Graphical LASSO

Friedman, Hastie, and Tibshirani have proposed a method to plot sparse graphs by a LASSO penalty applied to the inverse covariance matrix [22]. This method is called the *graphical LASSO* and has been implemented in the R package 'glasso' with remarkable speed using a blockwise coordinate descent algorithm. Speed is less important in the context I have been discussing, which is about 10–20 biomarkers and other variables, but the authors have shown remarkable speed of a simple and fast algorithm in higher-dimensional settings estimating approximately 500,000 parameters. The authors impose the L_1 penalty for estimating the Σ^{-1} matrix parameters.

The procedure cycles through the variables, fitting a modified LASSO regression to each variable in turn. The individual LASSO problems are solved by coordinate descent. Through various examples of synthetic and real data sets, it has been shown that the algorithm is able to produce the sparse topology of the estimated network of the data.

Using R package 'glasso', we can specify a regularization parameter vector for all edges (e.g., if certain edges are to be missing or always present, we can specify that also), or we can specify an overall regularization parameter for the graph.

23.1.3 Graphical Models via R Package 'qgraph'

The R package qgraph [23] integrates modeling, visualizing, and regularizing the partial correlation network in a comprehensive manner. A few things
to keep in mind about 'qgraph' discussion are as follows:

- Even though, Epskemp et al. have implemented networks of covariances, regression parameters, p-values, and other parameters, we
  will focus on the partial correlation network.

- Many visualization modes are available, we will however focus on
  the Fruchterman–Reingold (FR) algorithm.

- The package is able to model relationships between binary variables,
  continuous variables (GGM), or partial correlation network analysis.
  One of the great aspects of the integrated methodology offered by
  the package, 'qgraph' is the ability to have a mix of variables in your
  model. If you have a binary model in your network, qgraph uses the
  methodology provided by R package 'lavaan' to calculate polychoric
  associations between the ordinal and continuous variables.

- Another useful tool that is provided is if the correlation matrix is
  not positive definite, then other R packages are called to compute the
  nearest positive definite matrix before proceeding with regularization.

- Lastly, the LASSO procedure provided by the R package 'glasso' is
  used in 'graph'. A sparse Gaussian graphical model is computed by
  choosing a tuning parameter (see R code below). The tuning parameter is chosen using the Extended Bayesian Information criterion (EBIC)
  described by Foygel and Drton [24] in 'qgraph'. Choosing the tuning
  parameter as 0 makes no regularization or simply uses the BIC criterion, and choosing the value 0.5 yields the sparsest network. Choosing
  the parameter somewhere in between, say 0.25, usually works well.

23.1.3.1 R Code

```
Xy=read.csv("bmtrt.csv")
Xy=data.frame(Xy[,3:ncol(Xy)],y=Xy[,2])
X=Xy[,c(1:(num.biom+1))]
y=Xy$y
head(Xy)
library(qgraph)
cor_mat=cor_auto(Xy)
Cairo(file=file.path(loc,"Fig7.png"), type='png',
      width=5, height=5.5,units="in",pointsize=12,res=600)
qgraph(cor_mat,graph='glasso',layout='spring',sampleSize=nrow
(Xy),tuning=.2)
dev.off()
#Compare with reg
summary(reg)
```

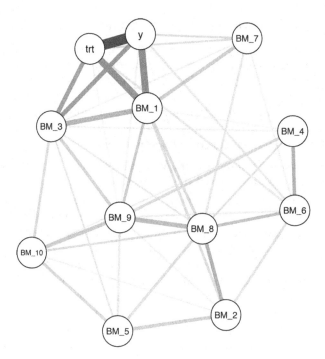

FIGURE 23.2
Graphical Lasso Correlation Network.

The 'qgraph' output gives the graph shown in Figure 23.2.

We see that strong edges are present between (i) treatment and the clinical outcome (negative association), (ii) treatment and biomarker 3 (negative association), (iii) treatment and biomarker 1 (positive association), and (iv) clinical outcome and biomarker 1 (positive association). These are true relationships, since I generated the synthetic data set.

The primary relationship between outcome and other covariates (first-order) are also detected by the regression model, which is contained in the object 'reg' for comparison.

The qgraph object can be stored in a variable and manipulated to produce the regularized correlation coefficients. This is a very useful feature indeed. I leave the reader to explore this package.

The 'glasso' algorithm does a pretty good job in detecting the most important associations (which may be predictive relationships) of the network of inter-relationships. It is a significant advantage to perform this type of multivariable in the setting of small sample size, since univariate hypotheses testing would be subject to multiple comparisons.

Some of the caveats to keep in mind for this analysis are as follows:

- the edges detected in the sparse network are subject to available sample size
- the absence of an edge does not mean there is no association between the two variables because the estimation dependent on what variables are in the model and the sample size
- the edge thickness does not measure the actual association between the two variables, since the model is regularized

References

1. McLeod AI, Xu C. (2018). bestglm: Best Subset GLM and Regression Utilities. R package version 0.37. https://CRAN.R-project.org/package=bestglm
2. Xu C, McLeod AI. (2009). Linear Model Selection Using the BICq Criterion. Vignette included in bestglm package, The University of Western Ontario.
3. Xu C, McLeod AI. (2010). Bayesian Information Criterion with Bernoulli prior. Submitted for publication.
4. Hastie T, Tibshirani R, Friedman J. (2009). *The Elements of Statistical Learning: Data Mining, Inference, and Prediction*, 2nd. New York: Springer.
5. Stone M. (1979). Comments on model selection criteria of Akaike and Schwarz. *J. Royal Stat. Soc.—Series B: Statistical Methodology*, 41(2):276–278.
6. Shao J. (1993). Linear model selection by cross-validation linear model selection by cross validation. *J. Am. Stat. Assoc.*, 88:486–494.
7. Friedman J, Hastie T, Hofling H, Tibshirani R. (2007). Pathwise coordinate optimization. *Ann. Appl. Stat.*, 1:302–332.
8. Draper NR, Smith H. (1998). *Applied Regression Analysis*. 3rd ed. Wiley.
9. Miller A. (2002). *Subset Selection in Regression*. 2nd ed. Chapman & Hall.
10. Tibshirani R. (1996). Regression shrinkage and selection via the lasso. *J. Royal Stat. Soc.—Series B: Statistical Methodology*, 58(1):267–288.
11. Zou H, Hastie T. (2005). Regularization and variable selection via the elastic net. *J. Royal Stat. Soc.—Series B: Statistical Methodology*, 301–320. doi:10.1111/j.1467-9868.2005.00503.x.
12. Lim M, Hastie TJ. (2015). Learning interactions via hierarchical group-lasso regularization. *J. Comput. Graph. Stat.*, 24:627–654.
13. Yuan M, Lin Y. (2006). Model selection and estimation in regression with grouped variables. *J. Royal Stat. Soc.—Series B: Statistical Methodology*, 68(1):49–67.
14. Lim M, Hastie T. (2019). glinternet: Learning Interactions via Hierarchical Group-Lasso Regularization. R package version 1.0.10. https://CRAN.R-project.org/package=glinternet
15. Straka P. (2019). *Add Interactions to Regularized Regression|Peter's Homepage*. Peter's Homepage. https://strakaps.github.io/post/glinternet/ [Accessed 3 September 2019].

16. GitHub. (2019). *topepo/caret*. https://github.com/topepo/caret/tree/master/ models/files [Accessed 4 September 2019].

17. Fruchterman TMJ, Reingold EM. (1991). Graph drawing by force-directed placement. *Software Pract. Exp.*, 21:1129–1164. doi:10.1002/spe.4380211102.

18. Kamada T, Kawai S. (1989). An algorithm for drawing general undirected graphs. *Inf. Process. Lett.*, 31:7–15. doi:10.1016/0020-0190(89)90102-6.

19. Jones PJ, Mair P, McNally RJ. (2018). Visualizing psychological networks: A tutorial in R. *Front. Psychol.*, 9:1742. doi:10.3389/fpsyg.2018.01742.

20. Dempster AP. (1972). Covariance selection. *Biometrics*, 157–175.

21. Pourahmadi M. (2013). *High-Dimensional Covariance Estimation*. John Wiley & Sons.

22. Friedman J, Hastie T, Tibshirani R. (2008). Sparse inverse covariance estimation with the graphical lasso. *Biostatistics*, 9(3):432–441.doi:10.1093/biostatistics/ kxm045.

23. Epskamp S, Cramer AOJ, Waldorp LJ, Schmittmann VD, Borsboom D. (2012). qgraph: Network visualizations of relationships in psychometric data. *J. Stat. Software*, 48(4):1–18. http://www.jstatsoft.org/v48/i04/

24. Foygel R, Drton M. (2010). Extended Bayesian information criteria for Gaussian graphical models. In Advances in neural information processing systems (pp. 604–612). https://papers.nips.cc/paper/4087-extended-bayesian-information-criteria-for-gaussian-graphical-models

25. Breiman L, Friedman JH, Olshen RA, Stone CJ. (1984). *Classification and Regression Trees*.

26. Therneau T, Atkinson B. (2019). rpart: Recursive Partitioning and Regression Trees. R package version 4.1-15. https://CRAN.R-project.org/package=rpart

27. Breiman L. (2001). Random forests. *Mach. Learn.*, 45(1):5–32. doi:10.1023/A: 1010933404324.

28. Kuhn M. (2019). Contributions from Jed Wing, Steve Weston, Andre Williams, Chris Keefer, Allan Engelhardt, Tony Cooper, Zachary Mayer, Brenton Kenkel, the R Core Team, Michael Benesty, Reynald Lescarbeau, Andrew Ziem, Luca Scrucca, Yuan Tang, Can Candan and Tyler Hunt. caret: Classification and Regression Training. R package version 6.0-84. https://CRAN.R-project.org/ package=caret

29. Bou-Hamad I, Larocque D, Ben-Ameur H. (2011). A review of survival trees. *Statist. Surv.*, 5:44–71. doi:10.1214/09-SS047.

30. Fu W, Simonoff J. (2018). LTRCtrees: Survival Trees to Fit Left-Truncated and Right-Censored and Interval-Censored Survival Data. R package version 1.1.0. https://CRAN.R-project.org/package=LTRCtrees

31. Chen B. (2017). A Package for Biomarker Threshold Models_. R package version 1.15. https://CRAN.R-project.org/package=bhm

32. Chen B, Jiang W, Tu D. (2014). A hierarchical Bayes model for biomarker subset effects in clinical trials. *Comput. Stat. Data Anal.*, 71:324–334.

33. Fang T, Mackillop W, Jiang W, Hildesheim A, Wacholder S, Chen B. (2017). A Bayesian method for risk window estimation with application to HPV vaccine trial. *Comput. Stat. Data Anal.*, 112:53–62.

34. 5 Amazing Types of Clustering Methods You Should Know—Datanovia. (2019). Retrieved 8 September 2019, from https://www.datanovia.com/en/blog/ types-of-clustering-methods-overview-and-quick-start-r-code/

35. Kassambara A, Mundt F. (2017). factoextra: Extract and Visualize the Results of Multivariate Data Analyses. R package version 1.0.5. https://CRAN.R-project.org/package=factoextra

36. Kassambara A. (2017). *Practical Guide to Cluster Analysis in R: Unsupervised Machine Learning* (Vol. 1). STHDA.

37. Hierarchical Cluster Analysis UC Business Analytics R Programming Guide. (2019). Retrieved 8 September 2019, from https://uc-r.github.io/hc_clustering

38. Morgan JA, Tatar JF. (1972). Calculation of the residual sum of squares for all possible regressions. *Technometrics*, 14(2):317–325. doi:10.1080/00401706.1972.10488918.

Section V

Biomarker Statistical Analysis Plan

Section 1: Introduction

In the introduction of biomarker Statistical Analysis Plan (bSAP), a clear and concise statement regarding the rationale for the biomarkers included in the study and their analysis should be laid out. This includes a description of the molecule (drug) and its mechanism of action, the therapeutic area, and the main clinical outcome. Overlap with the study protocol and main statistical analysis plan (SAP) should be minimal. The disease progression mechanism, drug action and the measured biomarkers should be described. If one or more biomarkers are for mechanism of action and target modulation, then that should be laid out. If there are markers for measuring or monitoring disease progression, then those should be introduced. If markers are being considered for predictive purposes or as surrogate endpoints, then that should be made clear. What is out of scope for the plan should also be mentioned. For example, a main predictive biomarker for enhanced treatment benefit may be addressed comprehensively in the main SAP for the clinical study protocol. The bSAP document will capture all supplemental analyses in this case.

This is simply a suggested format and it can be altered to suit your needs. For example, if your objective is to carry out comprehensive analysis of a single biomarker as a surrogate endpoint spanning data from one or more trials, then you would include that analysis here as the primary focus, or in the study SAP, or you can split the bSAP into two documents or parts: one for the surrogate endpoint analysis and another for the rest of the biomarkers.

The main objective is to give a framework for the results of the biomarker analysis for correct interpretation as exposure and/or effect and as a cumulative body of evidence in favor (or not) of the disease biology and/or drug action obtained through the clinical trial.

Section 2: Study Design

The study design should be described briefly. If necessary, the main visual or graphic for the design could be included here. The study protocol should be referenced. If the biomarkers played a role at any point in the study design, then it should be noted. For example, a predictive biomarker may be used to stratify entry into the study for patients.

Section 3: Biomarker Rationale

In this section, the names of the biomarkers must be listed under each type of biomarker. A few type of biomarkers may be

- predictive biomarkers
- prognostic biomarkers
- other disease-related biomarkers
  - which may measure severity or safety or may even be closely associated with the clinical outcome as a surrogate biomarker
- mechanism of action related
  - for example, mechanism of action type of biomarkers may include PET or MRI imaging, which leads to complex statistical analysis
- others

Note that if a biomarker is predictive and the cutpoint is known, then that type of analyses is usually contained in the main SAP of the trial. However, the statistician working on the biomarker plan, in conjunction with the study statistician, may lead the effort in finding the optimal threshold or doing multiple subgroup analyses. These are the cases where bSAP may be written with clear objectives specified in this section.

Clearly identify the biomarker(s) and why it is being measured, since this is a crucial goal of this part of the bSAP. The scientific rationale is the main idea to be covered in this section. Further specify when the biomarker is measured and relevant assessment schedules.

Section 4: Objectives

Typically, biomarker analyses will have multiple objectives in the trial. You could have multiple biomarkers in the trial for assessing (i) mechanism of action, (ii) prediction of clinical utility, (iii) disease monitoring panels, and so on. State the objective for each of the different types of biomarker(s). Typically, it would not be meaningful to classify the biomarkers as primary or secondary as the main SAP. If you have different types of biomarkers, it may be useful to break down the objectives by either type or the timepoint of the analysis.

For example, this is a list of objectives you might have

- To explore treatment-related changes in biomarker BM1, BM2, BM3, etc. at six months after initiating treatment in order to inform dosing or to understand disease progression
- To assess two additional cutpoints for predictive biomarker BM4 for efficacy outcome at 12 months
- To identify potential predictive biomarkers and their treatment interaction effects for biomarkers BM5, BM6 and BM7 at the end of the study
- To explore the direction and strength of interrelationships between a set of biomarkers values at six months of treatment
- To develop a 'responder' signature based on biomarker changes at month six of treatment
- To explore the timecourse profile of one more biomarkers and potential dose by time interaction of the trajectory
- To establish biomarker BM8 as a surrogate endpoint for clinical endpoint c in disease x
- To assess the safety profile of the treatment as determined by changes in biomarkers BM9, BM10, BM11 at six weeks

You can choose to group these objectives by time of analysis (baseline, six month analysis, and end-of-study analysis) or by type of biomarker analysis. Each group of objectives or subsections can repeat in the following section so it is easier to follow. For example, if you have a predictive biomarker in your objectives, then you will have a corresponding endpoint below for evaluating this objective. Alternatively, if your objective is to identify a cutpoint for a continuous biomarker, then state it as 'Cutpoint Determination'; carry through the same title for a subsection under Section 4 for endpoints.

It is sometimes useful to rank order any hypotheses testing within a group of biomarker objectives. If there is a testing strategy, it can be explained in Section 5 and/or 7.

If a biomarker data will be used to make go/no-go decision about the trial or select a dose then, it should be stated here. The decision-making criterion should be nailed down.

Section 5: Endpoints

For each biomarker, an endpoint needs to be declared in this section.
For example,

- Percent change from baseline at 6 months in biomarker BM1 will be compared between the treated and placebo groups. The time point of 6 months in this example should have been rationalized in the Objectives or the Rationale section above
- AUC between 0 and 12 months for biomarker BM2 and BM3 of the different dose groups
- Sensitivity, specificity, and overall accuracy for the 'responder' algorithm when compared with 12 months' clinical response in both treatment groups

Typically, the trial is not sized based on testing biomarker-related hypotheses; however, if any of the biomarker endpoints did play a role in sample size calculations, then that should be added as an independent section in this document.

If a prediction model is to be developed, which outputs a score or a binary output from multiple biomarkers as input, then that should be stated as well. For example, a 'responder' will be identified from these five biomarkers using a model or a criterion. The rule or criterion if known would need to be stated in Section 7, otherwise details of developing the model would need to be stated in Section 7.

Lastly, it is a good idea to mention the clinical endpoints of the trial as a recap in a subsection.

Section 6: General Considerations for Analysis

Define the *population of analysis*. There may be more than one, for example, the safety population may be used to search for a toxic signal using specific biomarkers.

Account *for multiplicity correction* if any of the biomarker hypotheses are to be tested in order or if there is FDR or FWER controlled error rates.

Missing data mechanisms to be used should be identified. For one or more biomarkers, the limit of detection may need to be specified and rules for when a sample falls outside the range. For biomarkers, missing longitudinal measurements, assumptions about MAR (missing at random) or MNAR (not at random) should be stated and proper imputation methods identified. Multiple methods can be investigated here as sensitivity analysis.

Data preprocessing and normalization steps should be described. This section can be broken out by technical types of biomarkers, for example, immunohistochemistry (IHC), circulating tumor cells (CTCs), RNA-Seq, flow cytometry, real-time quantitative reverse transcription polymerase chain reaction (RT-PCR), etc. Raw data and algorithms for preprocessing and normalizing should be described.

Data derivations and transformations should be explained up front here. Numeric values, or changes from baseline, or percent change from baseline, or fold change or further normalization by a reference value and adjusted by the baseline value are a few examples of derivations that might be needed for analysis. Similarly, log transformations or another type of transformation may be necessary for parametric modeling. The definitions and formulae, if applicable, should be mentioned.

Section 7: Statistical Methods

Statistical methods should be discussed in this section for each of the biomarker objectives and endpoints identified above. If the objectives were grouped, then the statistical methods can also be described in similar groups. For example, the analyses is grouped by time: six weeks' biomarker data analysis; six months' biomarker data; end-of-study biomarker data; then, the analyses could be grouped as such. Alternatively, if you had grouped your biomarker data by type, predictive, mechanism of action, safety, then the analyses could be grouped as such. Within each group, the objectives and endpoints may be ranked in order of importance.

The statistical methodology should be laid out in a concise manner keeping in mind some of these types of analysis mentioned below:

- Statistical tests of hypotheses should be specified in this section. Parametric and/or nonparametric models used must include a brief justification and appropriately referenced in the Appendix. If there is any multiple comparison procedure is used, then that should be stated along with the level of alpha being protected.

- Visual plots should be described so that it is easy to summarize treatment differences. Longitudinally collected biomarkers, for example, are often plotted as spaghetti plots, as well as with mean and SE, with linear mixed model repeated measures (MMRMs) model calculated parameters.

- Descriptive summaries as either plots or tables should be mentioned in this section as well. For dichotomous biomarkers, the definition of positive and negative needs to be specified here.

- For predictive biomarkers, the threshold(s) being considered or being optimized needs to be specified precisely. Subgroup testing depending on different cutpoint (threshold) values should be described in detail. The sequence of testing several hypothesis may be specified.

- Technical details of assays and diagnostic tests or engineering specifications of equipment are best specified in separate charters. This document can reference the charters needed for details. But, if additional normalization steps for the biomarker data analysis are necessary, then they can be mentioned in this section or in Section 6 in *Data preprocessing and normalization*.

- For biomarkers evaluating the disease progression and/or being used as a stand-in for the ultimate clinical outcome, the timepoints and analysis model must be specified here (for example, MMRM – mixed effect repeated measures model, or Cox regression model for time to event outcome, etc). Usually, these biomarkers are modeled separately from the clinical outcome, if joint modeling of such a biomarker and the clinical endpoint is necessary, because of measurement error, then the procedure would be described here.

- If multimarker algorithm is developed, the details should be captured here. For example, if a tree model is used, then it should be mentioned here. Multiple competing models can be used. Training and test set strategies should be specified, for example, a fivefold cross-validation loop will be used. Appropriate references should be listed in Appendix for the method. Programming languages and versions should be mentioned.

- Graphical models, if used, should be described here as well. This could be tied to an objective of exploratory analysis for inter-relationships between biomarkers and clinical outcome.

References and Appendix

References

Here all the references to study protocols, SAP, imaging, genomic or other charters, should be provided. In addition, all statistical references are mentioned here.

Appendix A: Programs

Common R code and functions in languages other than R, for making derivations, simulations, modeling, and testing, can be included here in Appendix for the biomarker programmer. For example, you can include the permutation procedure to derive the distribution of the maximal T-statistic statistic here.

Appendix B: TLG

Mocks of graphs and tables can be provided in another Appendix.

Appendix C: Visit Tables

The timepoints for collection of biomarkers and analysis timepoints can be included as a table for ease of reference.

Index

Note: Page numbers in italic and bold refer to figures and tables, respectively.

Printed in the United States
by Baker & Taylor Publisher Services